NHS is not WORKING

Dr. Hamid Sarwar

Second Edition with
Addition of a Brief Summary

dr.hs@nhsisnotworking.com

Second edition published by
Grosvenor Books, London 2019

Typeset by
Plusgroup Ltd, England

Printed in Great Britain
by Amazon

This book is dedicated to the exceptionally talented and devoted doctors and nurses of the NHS, who provide their patients with outstanding service, despite the 'autocratic top-down management' inflicted on them by the lay managers.

The deficiencies and negligent practices of the NHS described in this book are all due to the inefficiency, ineffectiveness and incompetence of the communist-inspired, centrally controlled management infrastructure.

NHS doctors and nurses are some of the best in the world.

If you are one of the four million people waiting to see a hospital specialist in 2018, you will understand physical pain and mental anguish, which is a repeated theme running through this book. If you are one of the millions of people unable to secure a prompt GP appointment, you will understand what this book is all about.

I address this book to the 60 million people or so in the UK who have not used the NHS, or who have only briefly used A&E, and are therefore unaware of the sufferings of those *waiting and waiting*. One day it could be you!

Acknowledgements

I would like to thank the NHS hospital consultants, junior doctors, nurses and GPs for their insights and contributions. I would also like to extend my gratitude to the hundreds of NHS users who were interviewed as part of my research.

I thank my friends Steve Bristow, without whom the entire project would not have materialised, and Shaun Hurley, for his invaluable advice. I am most grateful to my wife Chatto, for her support and intellectual contribution, and for the encouragement of my lifelong friends, Judy & Humphrey Scott-Moncrieff.

Author's special note

The constant stream of feedback from friends, mentors and editors, who were so shocked by some of the information provided in this book that they wanted to know if it was accurate, took me aback. I hereby declare that all the material presented is correct and true to the best of my ability. Here is a list of the sources I used during my research:

Adam Smith Institute
BBC
British Medical Journal
Care Quality Commission
Centre for Health & Public Interest
Commonwealth Fund
Competition & Marketing Authority
Clinical Commissioning Group
Education Policy Institute
Euro Health Consumer Index
EU Primary Care
Forbes
Full Fact
Health Foundation
House of Commons Library
Institute of Economic Affairs
Institute of Fiscal Studies
Institute for Health Metrics and Evaluation
King's Fund
Mental Health Foundation
Met Police
National Audit Office
National Institute for Health and Care Excellence
NHS Choices
NHS Commissioning Board

NHS Confederation
NHS Digital
NHS England
NHS for Sale
NHS Improvement
Nicholas Timmins
Nuffield Trust
Office for Budget Responsibility
Office for National Statistics
Patients 4 NHS
Peter Drucker
Private Health Advice
Public Health England
Pulse Magazine
Quality Watch
Reform
Royal College of Emergency Medicine
Royal College of Nursing
Royal College of Paediatrics
Royal College of Physicians
Royal College of Surgeons
Sky News
Social Market Foundation
The Commonwealth
The Daily Express
The Daily Mail
The Economist
The Guardian
The Independent
The Lancet
The Observer
The Telegraph
The Times
UK Public Revenue
UK Home Care Association
Wikipedia
World Health Organisation

With Smoke and Mirrors 'Not so Simple' Simon Stevens CEO *NHS England* Strikes Again

Having failed miserably to stop the decline of the NHS-Management with his 5 Year Plan in 2014, the CEO of *NHS England*, Simon Stevens, has come forward with a 10 Year Plan in January 2019. He has totally failed to understand that technological wizardry and 'digital doors' offer no solution to the agony of the people waiting for 6 months to see a hospital specialist and 8-12 months to have a surgical procedure. Nor can this delusion of the future, halt the perpetual insolvency of the NHS. My book has become even more relevant after seeing what Simon Stevens has to offer over the next 10 years and offers a solution.

After publication of the book in September 2018, the overwhelming feedback was that the generous supply of facts and statistics had manged to obscure the main message of the book.

I have produced this small 'Summary booklet', to exclude the statistical detail and provide the crucial essentials. Hope it clarifies and motivates you to delve in to the main text of the book. You may find chapters 3, 7, 10 and 17 of special interest.

Dr. Hamid Sarwar
January 2019
dr.hs@nhsisnotworking.com

A Brief SUMMARY of the Book

Everything should be made as simple as possible,
but not simpler. *Albert Einstein*

Summary Sections 1 & 2 of the book

Summary Point (SP) 1: The book has three sections. Section one, 'what is not working in the NHS' (chapters 1-5) Section two, 'why the NHS is not working' (chapters 6-10) Section three, 'how can the NHS be changed to 'Put Patients First' (chapters 11-16). Publication of the book had to be postponed to write chapter 17 to research huge concerns raised by the new health secretary Matt Hancock announcing "My GP is through the NHS on Babylon Health, it's brilliant". Our research concluded: ***Never before has a Health Secretary shown such ignorance of the Fundamentals of the NHS***.

Summary Point (SP) 2: In spite of some of the best doctors and nurses in the world, the NHS-Management has turned the National Health Service to 'The Waiting Health Service'. The main and repetitive message of the book is the unacceptable and third world type delay to access any of the NHS services. This book is the first to identify the mental anguish and physical agony of the people waiting to get medical attention as their symptoms deteriorate.

SP 3: At the time of writing in 2018, four million people are waiting five to six months to see specialists and an additional five to six months for surgical treatment. Wait to see a GP is 10-14 days.

SP 4: Almost one million patients a week are unable to get appointments with a GP. A total of 11.3% of patients were unable to get an appointment at all. This amounts to around 47 million occasions on which patients attempted but failed to secure help from their GP, forcing them to give up and turn to A&E.

SP 5: In a survey of 2000 patients, with mental health problems one in six had attempted suicide while awaiting an appointment. Four in ten said they had self-harmed and two third said their condition had deteriorated before appointment with a mental health professional.

Patients are routinely waiting for more than a year for hip, knee, cataract, hernia, gallstone or tonsil procedures.

An increasing number of patients are being refused 'funding' for knee and hip surgery. Almost, 1,700 requests for such operations were turned down in 2017, 45% more than the year before.

SP 6: To avoid sleep disturbance; don't read this at bedtime.

Prepared to be Disturbed: The NHS-Management has created deliberately, a two-tier health care system 'An Instant Access Private Hospital Sector' for the rich' and the agonising misery of waiting for the rest. If you can afford £180-£250, you need not wait to see a specialist for 5-6 months, you can see the same NHS consultant or her colleague this week in the Private Hospital. If you are rich, you need not wait to have a surgical procedure for 8-12 months on the NHS. You can have this op in a Private Hospital next week.

Prepare to be Shocked: The NHS-Management has been spending millions of pounds of taxpayers' money to ensure the continued commercial existence of the Private Hospitals. This is how.

The horrendous NHS waiting lists forces the rich to go privately thus bypassing the NHS queues and providing the business that private hospitals need to make a profit for their owners.

The NHS-Management provides FREE treatment to the patients whose private operations have been botched or who have suffered complications. As many as 6000 patients a year need NHS care after bungled treatment at a private hospital. Half of them, around 2500, are 'emergency' cases who have to be rushed to the nearest NHS hospital, using a 999-ambulance call.

Here comes the Bombshell; this is no Conspiracy Theory. The NHS provides its very own fully employed six-figure-salaried consultants with generous pension schemes to private hospitals to do all work.

Read my lips. Private hospitals do not employ a single specialist doctor; everyone is a <u>fully employed NHS consultant</u>.

The ill equipped 5 star medical hotels making hundreds of million pounds profit would collapse instantly without the full support of the NHS. **There is no such thing as a private hospital sector in the UK; it is a scam created by the devious NHS-Management at the expanse of British taxpayers.**

Summary Point 7: In spite of having some of the best doctors and nurses in the world, the communist system inspired central economy-controlled model of the NHS-Management will never work, no matter how much cash is injected in this bottomless pit. The NHS employs 1.7 million people. There is no country in the world, where so many civilians are employed by the state except the Red Chinese Army (2.3million) and US Defence (3.2 million).

Summary Point 8: Every superlative in the English language would not do justice to the inefficiency, ineffectiveness, wastage, ignorance and 'conflict of interest' practices of the NHS-Management.

The sprawling soviet style NHS-Management model, led by the Health Secretaries with no experience of how the universal healthcare systems work, no business acumen, no vision, no accountability, no fear of financial deficits, advised and administered by the incompetent CEOs, is not fit for purpose.

Summary Point 9: 'Each year 2,500 people die of breast cancer, who would not have died if they lived in Belgium. Each year 3,200 die from bowel cancer, who would not have died if they lived in the Netherlands. A further 3,200 die from strokes, who would not have died in Switzerland.

'If you add up all the cases where more people die prematurely in Britain compared with these 'average' countries, it comes to 17,000 deaths. This is appalling. It is certainly nothing for us to be proud of. When people in Britain say they admire the NHS, I have to stop myself from gasping and saying, 'Are you aware of how the NHS saves fewer lives than other systems?' *Professor Karol Sikora*

Summary Point 10: The NHS performs worse than average in the treatment of eight out of the most 12

common causes of death, including deaths within 30 days of having a heart attack and within five years of being diagnosed with breast cancer, rectal cancer, pancreatic cancer and lung cancer. It is the third poorest compared to the 18 developed countries on the overall rate at which people die, when successful medical care could have saved their lives.
Report Kings Fund. Health Foundation. Institute for fiscal studies. Nuffield Trust.
Please read chapter three for details.

Summary Point 11: Here are few examples of wastage of money by the breathtakingly incompetent NHS-Management:
The total private finance initiative debt to the NHS is over £300 billion for projects worth only £55 billion. £245 billion has been wasted swelling the coffers of private companies.

Staff sickness absence costs £2.4 billion a year – £1 for every £40 of the total NHS budget. Forty-five thousand employees call in sick daily, 15 days per employee per year. Staff sickness absence is 1.8 times higher than in the private sector. 98 NHS-Management non-medical staff members get paid more than the UK Prime Minister. Over 600 quango chiefs are on six-figure salaries.

In 2015/16, the NHS spent an estimated £3.7 billion on agency costs (locum doctors and nurses). The NHS spends millions of pounds a year to provide translation services in 123 languages.

Would you believe it? This isn't fake news, or a misprint. The NHS-Management paid £1,322.52

for a 400gm tube of cortisone cream costing £1.90 and £1,579 for a 500ml tube of moisturiser costing £1.73. One hospital paid £16.47 for a single pack of 12 rubber gloves that should have cost 35 pence. Another splashed out £21.86 for one box of plasters costing £1.68.

Summary Point 12: The perpetually insolvent NHS-Management had annual budget of **£147.5 billion** in 2017/18. Without insulting your intelligence: £ 1 million = £1,000,000.

£1 billion = £1,000,000,000. One thousand million £147.5 billion is a mind boggling £147,500,000,000.

To put this money in perspective, the GDP of 140 countries in a world of 192 countries, was less than £147.5 billion in 2018. The Bill Gates Foundation's total worth is £55 billion. Heathrow extension would cost 18 billion.

Summary Point 12: With the staggering amount of money at its disposal, NHS-management has the lowest number of doctors, nurses, MRI Scans, CT Scans out of all the EU countries.

Summary Section Three of Book

How can the NHS-Management be changed to 'Put Patients First'

The big story is not that the NHS needs more money to stay afloat, the real issue is that no one is prepared to recognise that it needs to be run differently if it is to survive.' BBC and Sky journalists:

Summary point 1: In England there are 150 or so hospitals, which are geographically placed to be able to cover a catchment area of 275,000 to 350,000 people and serve the entire population of England. Larger hospitals may provide services to a greater number of people and may have more advanced and specialised facilities to treat patients from neighbouring hospitals. Each NHS hospital is a 'centre of excellence' and has been so throughout the NHS history.

These hospitals have been providing outpatients, inpatients, surgical procedures, A&E and diagnostic facilities. And have doctors, nurses technicians that are unmatched by any such institution in the world.

Please note: Our initial recommendations apply to NHS-management in England, excluding Scotland, Wales & N. Ireland.

Summary Point 2: The existing centrally controlled communist system inspired NHS-Management model would be dismantled and decentralised. All the management functions would be devolved to 150 or so regional hospitals; each would become *The Local NHS Centre*. Demolition and abandonment of the current NHS-Management would mean an end to the sham internal markets, conflict of interest ridden CCG's and all the quangos.

Summary Point 3: NHS for us, operating from 150 or so local hospitals as *The Local NHS Centres*, 'of the local People, by the local People, for the local People', is our proposed new model.

Each *Local NHS Centre* would be registered as a charity and would function independently. Local captains of business and industry would be invited to become trustees, to provide expertise in various areas of finance and management.

Summary Point 4: *The Local NHS Centres* would review existing loans, staffing levels and service agreements and, where feasible, negotiate new contracts. One of the major changes would be the provision of GP services to the local community, thus reversing the existing dynamics of the NHS management structure.

The *Local NHS Centres* would use local businesses and companies to provide competitive services and improve the local economy. Every *Local NHS Centre* would produce its own cost-effective and efficient systems to cater to the needs of a small local community. Please read chapter 12.

Summary Point 5: The creation of *The Local NHS Centres* would transform the old, unworkable NHS-Management to the new model, **'NHS for us'** "of the local People, by the local People, for the local People."

Summary Point 6: The Ethos and Culture of the new model would be based on three Goals: *Zero Patients Waiting List, Zero Financial Deficit and excellent satisfaction level of the patients, doctors, nurses and staff with the* **'NHS for us'**.

Summary Point 7: The **'NHS for us'** would never be privatised, nor a complex European style Health Insurance system introduced. People are already paying for a number of the services. NHS Dentistry has never been free since 1951 and there are 3 compulsory bands to pay:

Band A: £21.60   Band B: £59.10   Band C: £256.50
GP Prescription charge for each item is £8.80.
Eye tests £21.30. Each contact lens £57.
Surgical brassiere £28.85. Abdominal Support
£43.60. Spinal Support £43.60. Stock Wig £71,25.
Partial human hair wig £188.70. Full human wig
£275.95. *These charges as from April 18*

Summary Point 8: The most radical & important
recommendation of the model **'NHS for us'** is that
everyone using any NHS service must pay a small
amount, which would be capped and would NEVER
be more than £8/week in a 12 months calendar year.

Spending patterns of the 'British household', as
provided by the Office for National Statistics (year
ending 2017):
Recreation & culture, £73.50/week.
Restaurant & hotels: £50.10/week
Clothing & footwear: £25.10/week.
Alcohol drink £11.90/week

Summary Point 9: We recommend three bands of
payment in the **'NHS for us'** model, every time a
service is used.
Band A: £10: GP Visit, blood test, X Ray, ambulance
call, minor walk in injury clinic, hospital bed charge
for each day for the first 4 days of the stay.
Band B: £20: A&E attendance, MRI scan, CT Scan,
Hospital bed charge for each day from day 5 of the stay.
Band C: £50: Any inpatient surgical procedure.

The maximum payment anybody would ever pay in
one 12 months period would be £8/week or £416/
year; CAPPED.

Summary Point 10: If a person in the 12-month period should consult the GP 8 times, calls an ambulance twice, visits A&E once, sees a hospital specialist once, has one MRI scan, one blood test, the total amount the person has spent is £170. An additional surgical procedure under General Anaesthetic would be £50. Add to it £40 for four days stay in hospital and the grand total for this almost maximum use of the NHS services in a 12 months period would be £260. Providing a conservative estimate, the cost to the **'NHS for us'**, for providing this set of services could be up to £5000 - £10,000.

Summary Point 11: A 'free-for-all' system creates unlimited demands and limits people from taking responsibility for their own health. The money paid for each service would contribute only a small amount of funds towards the **'NHS for us'** operational cost. The minimum cost of any NHS service is £100 and could be £1000-£10,000 or much higher.

Summary Point 12: For the first time ever, the **'NHS for us'** has a plan to achieve the 'Dual Miracle of zero waiting lists for patients and zero financial deficit.' Chapters 14, 15, 16.

Summary Point 13: One of the most notable discovery of the research of the book has been the obvious but unknown principal: "An insufficient number of doctors, nurses and diagnostic equipment would lead to an exponential growing waiting list, that no amount of reactive cash injection can solve. The only way to neutralise the awesome destructive power of the 'patients waiting list' on the entire NHS is to have enough number of doctors, nurses and diagnostic equipment". Chapter 14.

Summary Point 14: 'NHS for us' Regulatory Board, would implement the following actions:
1. In line with commercial companies, through a review of the contracts of employment, no doctor working full time or part time in the NHS can work for a private hospital or a private company which offers medical services. Such organisations would be required to apply for a licence, renewable yearly and employ their own doctors to operate and satisfy quality standards.

2. The GP's self-employment status would be abolished and changed to a salaried structure like their hospital colleagues. The recruitment of new GPs would be the job of **'NHS for us'.**

3. Every private hospital would require an annual licence to operate. This would be approved only if the hospital can prove its ability to operate as a stand-alone unit, mirroring every facility that an NHS hospital offers. Request for admission of a patient by a private hospital to an NHS hospital, due to whatever reason would lead to an immediate suspension of the licence.

Summary Point 15: Specially added, chapter 17 would explain why Matt Hancock's position as health secretary is untenable due to him declaring "My GP is through the NHS on Babylon Healthcare".
"Never before has a Health Secretary shown such

ignorance of the Fundamentals of the NHS". The company does not accept a patient if suffering from a list of 15 types of medical conditions.

Babylon's CEO Mr. Ali Parsa is the same gentleman who was going to revolutionise the management of the NHS Hinchingbrooke Hospital by the private company as CEO of Circle Holdings. The watchdog 'Care Quality Commission', for the first time in the history of the NHS, found the hospital to be "inadequate in all areas" and put it in special care. The ten years contract to manage the hospital was abandoned by Circle Holdings. The only beneficiary of this disastrous exercise was Mr. Parsa, who according to the Guardian was paid £1.1 million before he abandoned the sinking ship.

Conclusion: For the first time ever, this book has presented a blueprint to show that there is another way, a credible way, a workable way to change the perpetual insolvency of the NHS-Management and save the misery, anguish and pain of millions of people, suffering daily due to unacceptable delays to access any NHS service. The deteriorating morale of the people working under unimaginable stress and inevitable worsening standards of care due to shortage of doctors, nurses and diagnostic equipment must be reversed.

Please read this book to find out how the NHS-Management with some of the best doctors and nurses in the world can be changed.

The new model **'NHS for us'**, 'of the local people, by the local people, for the local people' would achieve zero patients waiting list and zero financial deficit.

In the first quarter of 2019, an extensive campaign would be launched by sending a hardback edition of this book to all the MPs, ministers, the PM, print media, radio and TV. Please help us to change what must be changed. If you are not one of millions of people suffering due to delayed access to the NHS today, please remember, you will need the services of the NHS one day.

I will be delighted to hear from you.
Dr. Hamid Sarwar

dr.hs@nhsisnotworking.com

NHS is not WORKING

Dr. Hamid Sarwar

Chapters

Prologue: Waiting for Godot *(Samuel Beckett)*

Chapter one: Some secrets are like fossils and the stone has become too heavy to turn over *(Delphine de Vigan)*

Chapter Two: You can fool all the people some of the time, and some of the people all the time, but you cannot fool all the people all the time *(Abraham Lincoln)*

Chapter Three: The Commonwealth Games

Chapter Four: "Is this a dagger which I see before me, the handle toward my hand?" *(William Shakespeare, Macbeth).*

Chapter Five: Waiting is like waiting for rain in drought. Useless and disappointing *(Hilary Duff)*

Chapter Six: Das Capital *(The Communist Manifesto)*

Chapter Seven: Grapes of Wrath *(Novel John Steinbeck; Bible Revelation 14: 19-20 new testament and Isaiah 63, old testament)*

Chapter Eight: Ground Control to Major Tom *(David Bowie).* Reforms so big, these can be seen from outer space *(Sir David Nicholson CEO NHS England 2006-2014)*
Balkanised Fiefdoms
(Jeremy Hunt, ex Health Secretary)

Chapter Nine: There are more things in heaven and earth, Horatio, than are dreamt of in your philosophy *(William Shakespeare, Hamlet)*

Chapter Ten: We are the hollow men, we are the stuffed men *(T.S. Elliot)*
Ask not what I can do for the NHS, ask what the NHS can do for me.' (US *President, John F. Kennedy 'ask not what your country can do for you- ask what you can do for the country')*

Chapter Eleven: If you don't know where you are going, any road will take you there *(Lewis Carrol, Alice in Wonderland)*

Chapter Twelve: A Farewell to Arms
(Earnest Hemingway)

Chapter Thirteen: A Tale of Two Cities
(Charles Dickens)

Chapter Fourteen: Corridors of Power *(C.P. Snow)*

Chapter Fifteen: A Paradigm Shift *(Thomas Kuhn)*
The first lesson of economics is scarcity; there is never enough of anything free of any value to fully satisfy all those who want it. The first lesson of politics is to disregard the first lesson of economics.
(Thomas Sowell)

Chapter Sixteen: Let us wake to a new dawn
(RN Tagore)

Chapter Seventeen: What can be cured must NOT be endured

Epilogue: Go Set a Watchman *(Harper Lee)*
Go, set a watchman, let him declare what he seeth
(Bible Isaiah 21:6)

Prologue

Waiting for Godot

This book is the result of extensive research and discussions with NHS hospital consultants, NHS hospital doctors training to be consultants, GPs and nurses. I worked in the NHS as a hospital doctor and general practitioner for over 20 years before making a career change.

I declare that I have no interest in a 'for profit' organisation, charity or similar. I have no affiliation with a political party or an ideological philosophy.

The National Health Service is now the 'waiting health service'. At the time of writing in 2018, four million people are waiting five to six months to see specialists and an additional five to six months for surgical treatment. Millions can't get a GP appointment for 11 to 13 working days. The NHS is commercially insolvent, in spite of a budget of £147.5 billion in 2017/18, which is more than the GDP of 140 out of 192 countries.

The main message of this book is:
You have no idea of the physical pain people go through as they wait for months to be seen or have an operation. You have no idea of the anguish people with mental health problems go through as they wait six to 12 months to see someone, often while feeling suicidal. You have no idea how it feels not to be able to get an

appointment to see a GP for weeks at a time when your child is ill. You have no idea how it feels to lie on a trolley in A&E for hours amongst dozens of people, as if it was a war zone.

This third world standard to accessing NHS services is unacceptable and must be changed.

We, the British public, have been brainwashed to believe in the 'miracle' of free NHS care and how the rest of the world suffers. Horror stories from the US reinforce this belief. The people of the UK know little of the better health services that the majority of EU countries offer their people. Inability to pay for access to any of these services is never an issue due to the Universal Healthcare System.

We will show the daily chaos, crises and near bankruptcy of the NHS. The slogans that read how it's the 'pride of the nation' and the 'envy of the world' exist only in the delusional minds of politicians and managers.

It is important for us to emphasise that the NHS has some of the most highly-trained doctors in the world, as well as excellent nurses. However, the NHS is not working because of its antiquated, communist-inspired management infrastructure.

Every superlative in the English language would not do justice to the inefficiency, ineffectiveness, incompetence, negligence, wastage, ignorance and conflict of interest practices inside the management of the NHS.

Strong words you might say, especially when you consider how the Conservative politician Nigel Lawson once described the NHS as 'the closest thing we have to a religion'. In subsequent chapters, I will prove to you what has been stated.

You will learn **what** is not working in the NHS, **why** it is not working and **how** can it be changed in order to **put patients first.** You will read about the secrets and scandals of the NHS that you never knew existed. Prepare to be amused, bewildered and shocked.

Apologies: My sincere apologies to the readers of this book with excellent memories. There are a few repetitive passages throughout, which has been done deliberately to convey the message.

Stop Press: The publication of the book had to be delayed to add the special chapter seventeen to research the implications of the new Health Secretary Matt Hancock, joining Babylon.

He declared "My GP is through the NHS on Babylon Health, it's brilliant".

Never before has a Health Secretary shown such ignorance of the fundamentals of the NHS.

SECTION ONE

What is Not Working in the NHS?

Chapter One

*Some secrets are like fossils and the stone
has become too heavy to turn over*

The founders of the NHS were aware of Marx
and Engels' provocative statement, 'History of all
hitherto existing societies is the history of class
struggle.'

The architects of the NHS aimed to ensure that by
providing a health service to the people of the UK,
the question of inequality (in terms of Karl Marx's
'bourgeoisie' and 'proletariat') would not exist.
How better to achieve this than by providing the
service free to everyone, so that no members of
the so-called 'bourgeoisie' would be given priority.
The concept of a 'free for all, equal for all' service
was thus presented to the nation.

Is it really 'free for all, equal for all'? Read this
account of a typical situation in a GP's surgery:

Patient: Doctor, the treatment performed by you
on my knee has not helped me for the last eight
weeks. I am now in pain all the time. Worst
of all, I am finding it impossible to work as an
electrician. You referred me to the specialist, Dr
Pennypound, in early February. I received an
appointment today but it's not for another six
months.

GP: Mr Shufflebottom, I am afraid there is
nothing I can do about it. You will have to wait.

Patient: I can't possibly wait that long. I cannot sleep at night. I find it so hard to work, but I cannot afford to be off sick, as I am self-employed with three children. Oh, doctor, please help. What can be done?

GP: Do you have private health insurance?

Patient: No.

GP: Are you prepared to part with £200?

Patient: I can't afford it, but I could arrange something.

GP: (Smile) Mr Shufflebottom, you can see the specialist, Dr Pennypound, PRIVATELY tomorrow morning – or please phone his secretary and tell her what time suits you.

Patient. Are you telling me, sir, that instead of waiting for almost six months to see Dr Pennypound on the NHS, I can see him privately this week by paying £200?

GP: Yes, that is correct.

Patient: I can't believe it. You thought that I might need an operation. What is Dr Pennypound's waiting list?

GP: His waiting list for an operation at our trust hospital is 20 weeks minimum, but it could be more. Some of my patients have been waiting for 26.

Patient: In other words, doctor, are you telling me that if I were to wait on the NHS, the total waiting period for my op would be almost 10 months or more? I couldn't possibly wait that long.

GP: You can go private. This could cost more than £6000.

Patient: Oh, that's a lot. I could consider cashing in the ISA that I have been paying into for ten years to give to my children, or I could remortgage my house. If I am able to raise this amount, when do you think I could have the operation privately with Dr Pennypound?

GP: (Broad grin). After seeing him tomorrow, you could have your operation next week!

The above drama is the type that takes place on a daily basis in every GP's consulting room. It is based on a true story, although, as you might have guessed, names have been changed. The total cost including the treatment, the first consultation, an MRI scan of the knee and the operation was around £7500. The patient in question took out a second mortgage on his house. He is now working full-time with no knee pain. He says the borrowed money was the 'best ever investment in his life'.

The NHS Secret Number One:
In the UK, we have a two-tier healthcare system: Private hospital sector for the rich; NHS for the rest.

If you have money or can beg or borrow some, you can see an NHS specialist in a private hospital this week. If you have money or can raise it, you can have an operation performed by an NHS specialist in a private hospital next week.

If you do not have the money, you will have to wait for five to six months to see the same NHS specialist (or his colleague). If you do not have the money, you will have to wait for an additional five to six months to have the operation.

Secret Number Two:
Let us revisit the creation of the NHS in 1948 by Aneurin Bevin. He faced fierce opposition from people such as the wealthy industrialist, Sir Bernard Docker, the eminent consultant, Lord Horder, and the secretary of the British Medical Association, Charles Hill. The entire medical profession was against it too. Bevin was described as a dictator and the few doctors who were willing to be a part of the new NHS were called 'quislings' (Quisling was the former head of the puppet government in Nazi-occupied Norway.)

Consultants were a formidable opposition, but Bevin overcame this hurdle by giving them more money. They were also allowed to keep their private practice whilst working in the NHS with full salaries. In Bevan's own and famously blunt words, 'I stuffed their mouths with gold.'

At the inception of the NHS, therefore, a small

parallel private health service was born. Instead of abolishing this unfortunate concession by Mr Bevin, politicians and NHS managers allowed it to expand.

Unknown to most, the NHS has spent large sums of taxpayers' money to produce a competing and parallel 'private hospital service'. I will show you how the NHS has achieved this. Over a period of 70 years, the National Health Service has been converted to a 'waiting health service': five to six months to see a specialist, an additional five to six months or more for having an operation.

No one in their right mind would pay to see a specialist or to have an operation if a free NHS was available without the horrendous waiting period. The 1976 Act of Health Services abolished private work from NHS hospitals, enabling a proliferation of private hospitals to spring up all over the country.

The NHS has been spending millions of pounds of taxpayers' money a year to look after the patients whose private operations have been botched or who have suffered complications. As many as 6000 patients a year need NHS care after bungled treatment at a private hospital. Almost half of them, around 2500, are 'emergency' cases who have to be rushed to the nearest NHS hospital.

Not one private hospital has an Accident & Emergency service; they have limited medical cover at night, no resuscitation teams, no intensive care or high dependency facilities. They all depend on the NHS to come to the rescue.

The 'private hospital service' is run from opulent, five-star private 'medical hotels'. None of these (except perhaps one or two in London) can survive as a standalone unit without the support of the NHS.

The majority of private hospitals would close if the NHS withdrew its free 24/7 support, which is paid for using taxpayers' money. These hospitals would also have to close if the NHS stopped sending its patients their way.

Contrary to the impression you may have, private hospitals derive only a small amount of their income from foreign paying patients, and most of these are in London. It appears that almost 99% of the income generated by private hospitals outside London comes from British taxpayers, directly or indirectly.

In 2015-2016, the NHS spent £8.7 billion on the treatment of its patients in private hospitals. The rest of the income comes from rich taxpayers busting NHS waiting lists.

Chapter Two

You can fool all the people some of the time, and some of the people all the time, but you cannot fool all the people all the time.

Please forgive me for repeating in brief the secrets of the NHS up to now. The UK has a two-tier health care system: a 'paying instant treatment' private hospital sector for the rich and a waiting National Health Service for the rest of the population.

You have learned that the private hospital sector was the masterful creation of the NHS. You have learned about the abolition of private work within the NHS by the Health Act 1976 and how decisions made by the NHS led to hundreds of millions of taxpayers' money being spent to provide free 24/7 help to private hospitals for botched operations and complications, which these glorified five-star medial hotels were simply not equipped to deal with.

As if this wasn't enough, here comes the bombshell.

Prepare to be shocked; this is not a conspiracy theory. The NHS provides its very own fully employed six-figure-salaried consultants to private hospitals to do all work.

Read my lips. Private hospitals do not employ a single specialist doctor; everyone is <u>a fully</u>

employed NHS consultant.

The provision of fully employed NHS specialists to work for the private hospital service is in direct violation of the internationally accepted 'Law of Conflict of Interest'.

It is a well-known fact that in public and private sectors, the person working for an organisation cannot work for a competitor.

The policy of the Met Police is strict and clear, stating, "the serving officers are not allowed to have business interests that mirror any form of policing activity or use specialist police skills or knowledge'.

Private hospitals do not have a single specialist in full-time employment; they are all NHS consultant employees on six-figure salaries and with lucrative pension schemes, generous holidays and study leaves.

The deceitful NHS has created, defying all principals of 'conflict of interest', a *Parasite* Private Hospital Sector. All the patients in these hospitals are seen and treated by the NHS consultants. The NHS provides free 24/7 support to these fancy, ill-equipped private hospitals, at the expense of the taxpayer.

This must constitute one of the greatest scandals of the 21st century.

The implications of this are huge. To start with,

it is clear that in reality the private health sector doesn't exist. It is a mirage, an NHS-created 'scam' (to put it mildly).Let us examine this 'scam' in more detail.

The NHS creates the horrendous waiting lists to access its services. The fear of waiting makes the rich take out so-called private health insurance. The British public suffers in silence while observing the presence of a scheme with only one aim:
'To help the rich to bust the queue of people waiting to see a specialist.'

In 2015, the net profit of private health insurance companies was £1.1 billion.

The NHS consultant, who is unable to see a patient for five to six months, is available at a private hospital consulting room at a cost of £180-250. The same surgeon would operate on a rich NHS customer next week in a private hospital, instead of the person waiting for 8-12 months from referral date. The NHS violates daily its motto of 'free for all, equal for all'

Let us repeat. There is no such thing as a private hospital sector. All patients are seen and treated privately by fully employed NHS consultants.

When you examine the creation of the so-called 'internal NHS market', the implications of the 'non-existent' private hospital sector are enormous. In an unbelievingly devious and scandalous way, the NHS is now able to divert its funds to the so-called private hospital sector. In simple terms, NHS managers allocate work to its fully employed specialists through ill-equipped private hospitals.

In 2015-2016, the NHS spent £8.7billion treating patients in private hospitals. Some of the private companies who own these hospitals increased their profits up to 100%.

Chapter Three

The Commonwealth Games

When a mother, desperate about her three-year-old daughter with a persistent cough, cannot get an appointment with her GP for 13 days.

When a man waiting to see a specialist spends five months unable to sleep due to pain.

When people with severe mental health problems are committing suicide because they are unable to see a psychiatrist.

When ambulances cannot gain access to A&E because there are so many others waiting outside.

When people are dying on trolleys in A&E.

When nearly every blind person is waiting 12 months to have a cataract operation.

When the NHS runs out of money year on year.

The NHS politicians and managers comment, *'The NHS has been judged the best, safest and most affordable healthcare system out of 11 countries analysed by the Commonwealth Fund.'*

What is this Commonwealth Fund? Is it a charity founded and funded by Commonwealth countries? No, not at all. It is a charity situated in the United States that has nothing to do with them. It's unclear why it would steal the name of Commonwealth to give the impression that it has. The Commonwealth is an intergovernmental organisation of 53 member states. The countries within it span all six inhabited continents, equivalent to 20% of the world's land area. In 2014, the GDP of the Commonwealth was $10.45 trillion, representing 17% of the world GDP when measured in purchasing power parity. The Commonwealth is an internationally recognised brand name that has nothing to do with a small charity situated in the United States of America.

Imagine a small British charity wanting to call itself 'Children's fund of America'. This would never be allowed.

The so-called Commonwealth Fund's findings are similar to when TV weatherman Michael Fish told the UK public that the forecast for the next 24 hours was fair and sunny, only for the country to be hit within hours by the worst storm in years. Rather than giving our opinion on what the misnamed charity says and what is the stark reality, here are the quotes from various publications:

Euro Health Consumer Index (ECHI):
'The NHS is only the 14th best of the health systems in Europe and is delivering mediocre results in too many areas of care, including patient survival. The NHS performance is inadequate in so many areas that it ranks just above healthcare in Slovenia, Croatia and Estonia. Too many patients wait too long to see a GP, get treated

in A&E and have a CT scan within a week for something serious like suspected cancer.

'The NHS denies cancer patients access to drugs that might extend their lives and fails to deliver improvements in quality of care made available by many other European countries.

'The NHS comes 28th out of 35 European countries for the number of doctors per 100,000 population.

'In the 11 years of assessing European countries, the NHS has never made it in the top 10 of the ECHI ranking. Sweden, Poland and the NHS are the worst among European healthcare systems, with poor accessibility. The NHS has autocratic top down management of a very skilled profession.'

Institute of Economic Affairs:
'The Commonwealth Fund report relies on highly subjective views and has no method of cross-country control. Because there is no split between funding and provision of medical services in the UK, the consumers and providers get their information from the same source.

'When the NHS is not going to provide a service/treatment, patients and the staff may not even be told about better ways of providing it. The NHS, thus, provides 'blissful ignorance'.

What is unusual about the Commonwealth Fund

study is that it is mostly based on inputs and procedures and not <u>outcomes</u>.

What would you make of a customer review of a coffee machine on Amazon, awarded five stars and praised to the skies, which then ended up by saying, 'the machine has just one minor downside, it has a poor record on making coffee. But otherwise it is fantastic and highly recommended'?

'NHS fails to prevent 5594 premature deaths every year, which could have been avoided with better healthcare.'

Theodore Dalrymple writing in the magazine *This Week*:
'The Commonwealth Fund report has produced a lot of publicity with no mention that thousands of people die every year in Britain who would have been saved in any other country in Europe.'

World Health Organisation:
'The NHS ranks 18th amongst the countries of the world.'

Adam Smith Institute:
'A report published by European Health Consumer Index, published the same year as the Commonwealth Fund report, ranks the NHS 14th amongst its competitors. We consider the EHCI report more credible because of its emphasis on patient outcomes. Comparing apples to apples, the NHS still ranks below average.'

Jessica Ormerod, from Public Matters
'It is difficult to square the Commonwealth Fund report with reality. The NHS is in crisis, with many hospitals regularly on black alert, routine operations cancelled, including cancer surgery, lack of provision of mental health services, a social care system that is collapsing and general practice in meltdown. The Royal College of Nursing has warned that the crisis is becoming the new norm.

'The bulk of the Commonwealth Fund report relies on a survey of patients and clinician experience and not clinical data.

'But, on what is arguably the most important measure of health outcomes, the NHS is next to US, at the bottom of the table.

'If the Commonwealth Fund does not consider health outcomes to carry any more weight than a patient satisfaction survey, how is it defining high performance?

'The health outcomes show that the Government and the NHS are letting the staff and everyone down. The idea of this report as a PR and vindication exercise should be rejected.'

The King's Fund
'The NHS performs poorly in terms of outcomes. The domains in the Commonwealth Fund report are not weighted, and because there are several areas of assessment, the UK's relatively good

performance in some of these swamps the effect of its disappointing outcomes.'

The Guardian newspaper described this paradox as, 'The NHS has only one black mark against it, its poor record on keeping people alive.'

The Global Disease Burden collaboration of academics (also known as the Institute for Health Metrics and Evaluation) looked at avoidable deaths across the world and found the NHS well behind most of Western Europe.

The NHS has fewer CT scanners – 8 per million – compared to the EU average of 21.4 and fewer MRI scanners – 6.1 million – compared to the EU average of 15.4.

The NHS has slipped down international league tables for infant mortality and is now ranked 15 out of a comparable 19 countries.

In a recent study of 195 countries, which assessed mortality rates from causes that should not be fatal if effective health care is in place, the UK is ranked 30th, similar to Malta and Portugal.

The *Independent* newspaper, quoting from the reputable medical journal *The Lancet*, said: 'The NHS has been ranked just 30th in a new global study.

'Experts analysed data on death rates over the last 25 years from each country, which they called the Healthcare Access and Quality HAQ Index.'

The Economist: 'About half of hospital trusts are forecast to be in deficit at the end of the financial year to the tune of £4 billion. Sanctions for those in the red are not exacting, providing little incentive to be thrifty.

'Britain ranks in the bottom quarter of the OECD, a club of mainly rich countries, when it comes to five years mortality rates for cervical and colon cancer. One reason is late diagnosis.

'The NHS is also something of a laggard in child health and has the ninth highest rate of infant mortality out of 33 OECD countries, a deterioration of about 10 places since 1990. Hospital admission rates in the NHS for asthma, a condition that can be treated in primary care, are 50% higher than the OECD average. The prevalence of neural tube defects are among the highest.

'Mental health takes up 25% of the disease burden of the NHS, but roughly 12% of the budget. A surgeon reports that in one hospital, budget cuts were so severe that there were no surgical pens to mark which bit of a patient to cut up.'

Professor Karol Sikora, Dean of the University of Buckingham and the Medical Director of Proton Partners International:
'Each year, 2,500 people die of breast cancer, who would not have died if they lived in Belgium. Each

year, 3,200 die from bowel cancer, who would not have died if they lived in the Netherlands. A further 3,200 die from strokes, who would not have died in Switzerland.

'If you add up all the cases where more people die prematurely in Britain compared with these 'average' countries, it comes to 17,000 deaths. This is appalling. It is certainly nothing for us to be proud of. When people in Britain say they admire the NHS, I have to stop myself from gasping and saying, 'Are you aware of how the NHS saves fewer lives than other systems?"

Abstracts from a June 2018 report produced by the Health Foundation, Institute for Fiscal Studies, The King's Fund and the Nuffield Trust:

'The NHS performs worse than average in the treatment of eight out of the most 12 common causes of death, including deaths within 30 days of having a heart attack and within five years of being diagnosed with breast cancer, rectal cancer, pancreatic cancer and lung cancer.

'It is the third poorest compared to the 18 developed countries on the overall rate at which people die, when successful medical care could have saved their lives, known as amenable mortality performers.

'It has consistently higher rates of death for babies at birth or just after and in the month after birth; seven in 1000 babies died at birth or in the week afterwards in 2016 compared to an average of 5.5 across the comparator countries.'

The researchers commented, 'the NHS is a perfectly ordinary service.'

Our comments:
It was a matter of shame and of huge distress to thousands of women and their families to hear the announcement in 2018 that since 2009 (for nine years), an estimated 450,000 women between 68 and 71 were not sent appointments for breast cancer screenings. It is thought that up to 270 women may have had their lives shortened as a result.

Following a late bowel cancer diagnosis, Andrew Lansley, a former Conservative health secretary, admitted that his 2010 programme of early bowel cancer detection had still not been implemented in 2018.

An NHS investigation in May 2018 found that 'failure to provide adequate, safe and prompt care contributed to the deaths of 13 patients with learning disabilities'.

It is time that NHS politicians and managers stopped playing the 'Commonwealth Games' via a report which has nothing to do with reality (and which has the CEO of NHS England, Simon Stevens, as one of its directors).

Chapter Four

Is this a dagger which I see before me,
the handle toward my hand?

The very first point of contact of someone seeking medical attention is the General Practioner, who historically has been treated badly by the NHS policy makers in the UK up to 2004.

Here, a GP who retired in 2003 recounts his working life within a four-person group practice: "The four of us had our own nominated patients, and I knew most of them personally. I saw some children grow up to become young adults and several adults reach retirement age. I knew every member of a family. If I was on holiday for a week, my patients would sometimes wait for me rather than see one of my colleagues.

'Our contract of employment obliged us to look after our patients 24/7. The surgery hours were 8:30am to 6pm. All partners had patient consultations twice a day – 10 sessions in all. One day was a half-day. There was always a Saturday morning surgery. One of us would then be on call over the weekend until 8:30am on Monday.

'Life was tough and sometimes unbearable. The greatest stress was the house visits. Registered patients could call the surgery and demand one. In my experience and that of my colleagues, more than 90% of house visits were trivial and doctors were used because transport was not available and/or to avoid paying a taxi fare.

'I will never forget a disturbing experience regarding a colleague who worked over a weekend. Come Monday morning, he did not look well. We used to meet for coffee at the end of our morning session and I saw him sitting in a corner holding his head. This is what he said: "I made 20 house visits over the weekend: two on Saturday night and three on Sunday night. I have had very little sleep in the last 48 hours. I am exhausted, and with a list of six more house calls today, I feel like killing myself right now. I can't carry on being used as a taxi driver and catering to the most trivial medical problems. It's humiliating!"

He then burst out crying. He was a highly intelligent and sensible person. I stood motionless. His story, which I could relate to, had a profound effect on me and brought on my own tears.

'The following year, the young doctor was subjected to a long and stressful investigation after he refused to visit a child whose mother had insisted on trivial house visits in the past, and instead offered her a surgery consultation. The child was diagnosed with meningitis and hospitalised.

'When a private company came to our city offering out of hours care for the patients at night and at the weekends, we immediately joined after gaining permission from what was then called the 'Family Practitioner Committee'.

'The responsibility to look after our own patients was significant. The on-call doctors referred the patients back, and we saw almost every patient who had been seen by the duty doctors at the next surgery session. No patient could be seen in the A&E department without a referral note from their GP, unless it was an accident or similar. Every patient requiring a hospital admission during the day needed to have a conversation with the admitting hospital doctor, and a referral letter from the GP was mandatory.

'I understand that nowadays patients must wait up to two weeks to see their GP. This could never happen in my time. We would be subjected to dozens of house calls, both after hours and over the weekends, if we made people to wait for an appointment. We still had to carry out a certain amount of night duties and suffer the trauma of being constantly in demand for house visits.

One night, I had a phone call at 1am for a house visit because "the baby was very ill and crying all the time". It was snowing outside, and I did not know the directions to the house. In those days, there was no sat nav. With a map in one hand, I drove and drove. The street names were covered in snow. Ultimately, I found the house and knocked, as there was no bell. After a few minutes, the door opened, and a young woman opened the door. She shouted, "You have taken a f****** long time to arrive, haven't you? The baby is asleep now." Then she slammed the door shut in my face.

'I stood frozen, both physically and mentally. Would I be treated like this if I were a plumber asked to repair a leak? The conversation with the colleague who wanted to kill himself flashed in my mind. From then on, the joy of working was gone, and I began to resent every house call. That year I took early retirement at the age of 55."

The period in the history of the NHS General Practice up to 2004 was a shameful example of exploitation and cruelty. How could a doctor be expected to offer services to the patients 24 hours a day and seven days a week? The most humiliating thing was that anyone could ask for and insist on a house call and the poor GPs had a list of 4-6 house visits every day. This number could be increased to 8-12 in winter. Several house call requests came after 6 pm and over the week ends. A vast majority of these requests for house visits were for trivial problems and GPs were used as 'free medical delivery drivers'.

There were instances of 'calling the quack' to visit by an offspring to prove the love to the mother, who had not been seen for months!

Mercifully, the Tony Blair Labour Government, decided to relieve the GP's from this misery and they were awarded a new contract, absolving them from availability after 6 pm and over the week ends. The rights of patients to aggressively demand house visits (are you 'bloody' coming to visit my grandma or not?) were severely curtailed.

Unfortunately, in keeping with the glorious traditions of the NHS managers, they failed to plan how to provide the week end and after-hours facilities to the patients. The attempted efforts to do it through badly trained,staff (currently111) have proved very unsatisfactory.

Recently the press has been highly critical of the way general practice is being managed by the NHS. According to the doctor's magazine Pulse and reported by the Times:
"The average wait to see a GP is two weeks. One practice in six has turned away patients seeking routine appointments in the past year, a survey has found."

Doctors told researchers they were offering appointments only for emergencies after finding they had no routine appointments available for four weeks. Nearly 17% of GPs said they stopped routine appointments at some point in the past year.

The Daily Telegraph reported:
"Almost one million patients a week are unable to get appointments with a GP. NHS statistics show that a total of 11.3% of patients were unable

to get an appointment at all. This amounts to around 47 million occasions on which patients attempted but failed to secure help from their GP, forcing them to give up and turn to A&E.

A survey of more than 800,000 patients found worsening access to family doctors, with patients increasingly giving up their search for help, even though their health was deteriorating.'

Please note these statistics are national and an early appointment with your own GP does not make this information wrong.

Our researchers were told that in several general practices, people are asked to ring at 8am for an appointment, only to be told at 10am after constantly engaged lines."

"Please ring tomorrow as we are fully booked today. No, we cannot give you an appointment for tomorrow or any other day. Try again tomorrow."

Before we start to criticise the UK GPs for their inability to offer prompt appointments, we need to explore the reasons for it.

There is reported a reduction in the number of GPs between 2010 and 2015.Between 2015 and 2017, the NHS allowed the number of GPs to decline further by 4.8%. The total reduction between 2010 and 2017 could be as high as 7%. During this period, the UK population increased from 63 million to 66 million (almost 5 %)

We wanted to know, why on average, the waiting time to see a GP had shot up to 11-14 days and, in some practices, even three weeks. Our researchers were told that there is only a certain amount of work, any person can do. If the maximum number of patients that can be seen in one consultation session is 20 and the demand is consistently for 30, waiting list would inevitably build.

This argument makes sense considering the reducing numbers of GPs, increasing population and escalating demand created by the internet search engines. Rapid deterioration in access and quality of afterhours and weekend GP service, provided by the notoriously inefficient, **111** through poorly trained non-clinical people has aggravated matters further.

Unable to access prompt GP services, people flock to the A&E department for what is basically a primary care matter. This has a significantly destabilising effect on rest of the operational structure of the hospitals. Those who should be seen by their GPs are now crowding A&E, making genuine emergencies wait on trolleys. We will be discussing this in more detail in forthcoming chapters.

Unfavourable coverage of the NHS General Practice by the media has further tarnished its reputation. According to one newspaper headline

"Thousands of patients have cancer diagnosed in A&E because they have not managed to see a GP, a study has found."

Flustered by the adverse publicity relating to GP appointments,the Head of the Royal College of General Practitioners said:

"'People should treat themselves, look up their symptoms and go to a pharmacy before phoning up their GP."

This statement became the subject of much criticism and the media pointed out that Primary care is a person's first contact with a doctor when they're seeking prompt medical attention. Was self-diagnosis being advocated?

The GPs did not help matters either, when 250 doctors at the annual British Medical Association conference in Bournemouth agreed this as a proposed new policy:
"Let us turn away the patients if we are too busy."

As the problems arising from GP appointments were making headlines, the NHS managers have come forward with an innovative idea.

The NHS is now in the process of allocating £45 million to a ludicrous scheme to train receptionists to be 'care navigators'. Their function would be to ask, 'Why do you want to see the GP?'

We have no idea how these 'care navigators' are going to discourage patients concerned about their health to seek a GP appointment. Primary care is the ability of a person to have an easy and quick consultation with the doctor, so that where required a referral is made to a specialist for early diagnosis and treatment.

Contradicting all the traditional practices of primary care, GPs in the UK are being told to slash hospital referrals. In controversial plans to cut costs, the NHS is rolling out a pilot scheme that will require GPs in England to seek approval from a medical panel for all non-urgent hospital referrals. This covers GP requests for scores of procedures, including hip and knee surgery, eye cataract operations, X-rays and scans. GPs won't be able to send patients to hospital without permission from a panel of other doctors.

This so-called 'peer review' scheme is being expanded nationwide, following a testing period in two North East regions. Our research indicates that *NHS England* has told health trusts to carry out weekly reviews of referrals from GPs within a short period. The NHS is offering financial incentives to Clinical Commissioning Groups to set such schemes, which aim to save money by slashing referrals by 30%.

An entire chapter could be written on this preposterous scheme and the bankruptcy of ideas of those running the state monopoly NHS. This indicates lack of trust in the professionalism of GPs, who are being told they don't know what they are doing. Yes, they could be paid a six-figure salary but, erm, they are so incompetent that they require 'cleverer' doctors to tell them how to practice correct medicine, and who to refer for an X-ray, scan or a second opinion from a specialist.

Our research indicates that no GP consultations have taken place to implement these reforms. In plain words, GPs are being told, 'You may be OK at treating colds and sore throats and prescribing painkillers, but you are not good enough to make decisions about anything else. We, the state, will tell you: 'Now, shut up, we don't want to hear any complaints. We don't think your opinion is necessary.'

This kind of insulting attitude by the NHS managers to the highly skilled GPs is not exactly boosting their already deteriorating morale.

The ostensibly regulated NHS General Practice system appears now to be a moneymaking machine for 'entrepreneur GPs'.

You may be interested to read the list of Britain's highest earning GPs in 2015–16:

Number of GPs	Drawings
One GP earned	£700,000–£799,000
Four GPs earned	£400,000–£499,000
11 GPs earned	£300,000–£399,000
193 GPs earned	£200,000–£299,000

Please note that GPs making such large sums are in minority.

We conclude that a **GP Service** that (1) makes people wait for 11 to 13 days after they have tried for hours to get an appointment, (2) offers no quality access after 6pm and over the weekends, (3) allows its doctors to work for private companies to provide instant appointments, (4) allows the greedy to make up to £800,000 a year, could be considered as one of the worst.

Chapter Five

Waiting is like waiting for rain in drought, useless and disappointing.

Both the PM, Theresa May, and the outgoing health secretary, Jeremy Hunt have made eloquent speeches about the trendy topic of mental health without taking the slightest action to reduce the 'killer' waiting period to access mental health services.

Some facts:
A report from the 'We Need to Talk' warns that the consequent delays in accessing treatment can be disastrous for patients. In a survey of 2000 patients, one in six had attempted suicide while awaiting an appointment. Four in ten said they had self-harmed and two third said their condition had deteriorated before they had a chance to see a mental health professional.

Children are waiting up to 18 months for mental health treatment.

The NHS is to blame for 400 suicides a year due to their failure to get a grip on the mental health problem epidemic, a shocking report reveals. (This report appeared in the *Mail on Sunday*, February 14th, 2016 by Glen Owen & Michael Blackley.)

The Guardian investigated and found 271 deaths between 2012 and 2017 after 706 failings by health bodies. In 2016, the same newspaper stated that the number of deaths among mental health patients has risen 21% in the last 3 years – from 1,412 to 1,713.

MP Norman Lamb said that the overall number of serious accidents involving 'avoidable deaths' has climbed 34% to 8139 per year

Young women have become almost invisible in the NHS Mental Health Policy, despite soaring levels of female suicide (which has doubled in recent decades) and self-harm (tripled since 1993).

In 2017, more than a quarter of children referred to specialist mental health services were turned away.

At any one time, one sixth of the population in England aged 16-64 has a mental health problem. While 23% of NHS activity is taken up by mental illness, in recent years, mental health trusts have received approximately 11% of funding.

A recent British Medical Association investigation has 'warned' that thousands of patients are waiting for more than six months for access to talking therapies. The British Medical Association made requests under the Freedom of Information Act to the 207 Clinical Commissioning Groups and 54 NHS mental health trusts regarding waiting times for accessing talking therapies. Of the 183 Clinical Commissioning Groups that replied, nine out of ten did not record waiting times, while 22 out of 47 responding from mental health trusts also did not keep any records. Of those who did keep records, the British Medical Association found 3,700 people waited for more than six months and 1,500 for more than a year. The longest waits were in Leicestershire, where patients waited for two years. In Essex and Derbyshire, people waited for a year and a half.

The disastrous NHS Mental Health Service is not working.

NHS England admits that four million people were on an NHS waiting list in early 2018. Considering that the population of England is around 55 million, that's almost one person in 14 on such a list. Unfortunately, the figures do not give an idea of how many of these people are awaiting elective surgery and how many will have their first assessment carried out by a surgeon or a physician.

The NHS has long abandoned its third-world-country-type target of seeing people within 18 weeks of referral.

Sophie Borland, a health editor for the *Daily Mail* says:
'Figures obtained through Freedom of Information show patients are routinely waiting for more than a year for hip, knee, cataract, hernia, gallstone or tonsil procedures.'

Professor Sir Mike Richards, the chief of the CQC (Care Quality Commission) believes that the model of acute hospital care cannot continue to meet the needs of today's population.

Patrick Carter, the ex health secretary Jeremy Hunt's adviser, expressed the view that hospitals are in a 'state of war'.

The number of people who attended A&E per day in 2017 in England was 64,782 on average. This means that in 12 months, 23,645,430 people out of a total population of 55 million attended A&E. In other words, 43% of the entire population in England visited an A&E unit.

The former health secretary Jeremy Hunt made the following statement in 2013:
'The winter is going to be tough, that's why the government is acting now to make sure patients receive a great, safe service, even with the added pressures the cold weather brings. This is a serious problem which needs fundamental changes to equip our A&E in the future.'

The former health secretary proudly announced that a sum of £250 million was being allocated to tackle this issue.

In December 2017, more than 20,000 patients were left waiting in ambulances outside A&E in just two weeks, new NHS data has revealed. The figures from Public Health England told how 4014 people were stuck in ambulances for more than an hour and 50 ambulances were diverted because A&E departments were full.

In January 2018, tens of thousands of non-urgent operations and procedures in England were cancelled and deferred due to winter pressures in A&E. The move prompted Jeremy Hunt to apologise to patients.

Dr Nick Scriven, from the Society for Acute Medicine, said, 'Delays at the front door can be life threatening. Several hospital trusts reported an overall bed occupancy of 94.5% due to huge surges in emergency A&E admissions. This is well above the safe standard target of 85%.'

In January 2018, a senior A&E consultant said, 'I personally apologise for the third-world conditions of the department due to overcrowding.'

Our interview with several A&E consultants revealed a general consensus that more than 35-40% people attending A&E could have been dealt with by a GP. The once prestigious A&E unit has now turned into an out of hours general practice same-day treatment centre.

Jeremy Hunt famously said in 2014: 'I have taken my children to A&E rather than waiting to see a GP.'

In the eight years since 2010, the number of people waiting for more than four hours for treatment in A&E rose by 600%.

Several observers visiting A&E departments

have compared scenes similar to World War Two casualty units; dozens of people lying helplessly on trolleys and writhing with pain for hours, with a few sobbing.

Figures show that only 4% of people with broken hips get pain relief within an hour. More heartrending to learn is that 12% of children in severe pain with fractures and 28% with moderate pain get no relief at all. According to the Royal College of Emergency Medicine, this kind of suffering inflicted on a child can cause permanent mental scarring.

Professor Russell Viner, president of the Royal College of Paediatrics, states that the NHS child mortality rate is amongst the worst in Europe.

The most worrying recent development in the provision of hospital services is the implementation of rationing, which is reminiscent of the communist era. In Chapter 4, we provided examples of devious practices where NHS managers have tried to ration GP services.

According to a recent report by the British Medical Journal, an increasing number of patients are being refused 'funding' for knee and hip surgery. Almost 1,700 requests for such operations were turned down last year (2017) – 45% more than the year before.

Ian Eardley, senior vice president of the Royal College of Surgeons, said, 'Hip and knee surgery has long been shown to be a clinically and cost-effective treatment for patients. We are therefore appalled that a number of commissioning groups are now effectively requiring thousands of patients to beg for treatment.'

The BMJ said there was emerging evidence that more patients were going private. The 'for profit' hospital group Spire reported a 12% rise in revenue from self-paying patients.

Who performed these operations? Yes, you have guessed it right, the full-time employed NHS surgeons!

Our research shows that the super quango NHS England, in pursuit of cutting vital medical services, has now come forward with the idea of refusing to offer surgical treatment for 15 clinical conditions, to include treatment for piles and varicose vein surgery. Apparently, there appears to be no benefit to providing surgical treatment for these conditions, but the NHS would save around £300 million in the process. The consultations are taking place between July 4th and September 28th this year (2018). If successful, rich patients would be able to have the treatment from 'for profit' hospitals.

NHS hospital services, forcing people to wait for up to six months causing unimaginable pain and misery to millions of people are not working.

SECTION TWO

Why the NHS is not working

Chapter Six

Das Kapital

Marx and Engels advocated in *The Communist Manifesto*:
'The proletariat will use its political supremacy to centralise all instruments of production in the hands of the state.' The system is called 'command economy' and the NHS is a classic example of it.

In the centrally planned 'command economy', the state makes economic decisions and controls what is produced and managed. This model assumes that only the state (or government) can work in the best interest of the people, and that the state needs to make decisions to meet social and national objectives.

This kind of 'central planning' is associated with Marxist-Leninist theory, the former Soviet Union and, more recently, Cuba and North Korea.

History shows us that enterprises controlled and managed by the state in democracies do not work. Aneurin Bevin, one of the architects of the NHS, said, 'A free health service is pure socialism and, as such, it is opposed to the hedonism of capitalist society.'

In 'command economy', everyone is employed by the state and the NHS has retained this glorious tradition.

According to Forbes, there is no country in the

world where a government employs more people than the NHS – 1.7 million people (excluding the non-government employers Walmart and McDonald's).

In the number of people it employs, the NHS is beaten only by the Chinese Liberation Army (2.3 million) and the US Department of Defence (3.2 million).

Such vast numbers of state employees may be suitable for two large armies, but, logistically, not to provide daily health care in the fifth largest economy of the world in a country of 65.5 million people. The UK's public is made to believe that it is patriotic to praise the NHS and that people in the other parts of the developed world are probably dying due to lack of medical attention. This is <u>not</u> true. All EU countries offer a 'Universal Health Care System'.

Peter Drucker, the late, world-famous American management consultant, educator and author, concluded:
'The two vital components of a successful enterprise are efficiency and effectiveness. Efficiency is doing the 'things right'. Effectiveness is doing the 'right things'. Without efficiency, the enterprise would wither and die; without effectiveness, there is no hope of survival.'

Effectiveness involves foreseeing the future trends and challenges of the enterprise. The 'command economy' has no understanding of how a commercial enterprise works. The NHS model is both 'inefficient' and 'ineffective'. It neither does the 'things right' nor 'the right things'.

For several years, the NHS has been spending more money than the budget would allow. In 2016, the National Audit Report Office showed that 238 NHS trusts were in deficit the previous year – an overdraft of £2.45 billion. Had it not been constantly propped up by the state, the NHS would have gone bankrupt decades ago.

The confused and confusing management structure of the NHS is naturally baffling. There are 209 clinical commissioning groups, 135 acute non-specialist trusts (including 84 foundation trusts), 17 acute specialist trusts (including 16 foundation trusts), 54 mental health trusts (including 42 foundation trusts), 35 community providers (11 NHS trusts, six foundation trusts, 17 social enterprises and one limited company), 7454 GP practices, 10 ambulance trusts (including five foundation trusts), 853 independent organisations providing care to the NHS patients from 7331 locations.

(The above information is from the NHS Confederation website 2017. The number of CCGs has since reduced and there is a possibility of other minor changes in figures.)

One can imagine the impossibility of managing

this complex structure, which is the result of each government trying to implement changes to this dinosaur since 1948, leading to what we have today.

There are more than 600 health quango chiefs on six-figure salaries amid NHS cash crises. Ninety-eight staff members get paid more than the UK's Prime Minister, up from 48 in March 2017. When the NHS deputy medical director was suspended on a full salary under suspicion of voyeurism, he was on £215,000.

Many of these expensive organisations are new structures, set up in 2013. Public Health England has 244 managers on six-figure salaries. PHE has 4,973 staff members and has spent almost five million on communications alone.

NHS Improvement has 102 employees – 79 officials on six-figures salaries with one person on £215,000. Their revenue budget was 172.2 million and not one pence of this was spent on doctors or nurses treating the patients in the wards or hospitals.

NHS Health Education England, created in 2012, has 43 managers on six-figure salaries, with their chief on £210,000.

These guys, who are earning more than our PM, regularly make speeches on the 'shortage of NHS funds'. No one knows why these people are on such high salaries and what 'evidence-based contributions' their organisations make while the NHS is struggling financially.

Hundreds of practices, good or bad, originate from one principal – good or bad. The unfortunate problem with NHS politicians and managers has been that for the last 70 years they have been changing practices without changing the principal, which is the fundamentally flawed NHS model. The NHS has been trying to play hockey with a golf club, which can never work, no matter how many changes you bring in the shaft or the face of said club.

According to the charity Full Fact, the NHS annual spend for 2017/18 was as follows:

Country	Total Expenditure	Expenditure per person
England	£122 billion	£2200
Scotland	£13.2 billion	£2500
Wales	£7.3 billion	£2300
N. Ireland	£5 billion	£2700

Total: £147.5 billion

This amount is staggering. Without insulting your intelligence, one billion pounds is £1000,000,000 – one thousand million pounds.

Multiply this sum by ten and you get 10 billion pounds.
10 x 1000,000,00 = £10,000,000,000.

Now please try to imagine £147.5 billion.

£147.5 billion = £147,500,000,000

The NHS's expenditure of £147.5 billion, which is increasing every year, is so huge that it belies the imagination. To put this amount in perspective, in 2018, the GDP of 140 countries out of a total of 192 was less than the expenditure of the NHS in 2017/18. Please note that we are talking here about the GDP and not the annual total budget of a country.

The Bill & Melinda Gates Foundation, which people think is going to change health care in developing countries, has a net worth of £55 billion (not £55 billion every year!). The controversial Heathrow airport extension would cost around £18 billion (and not every year).

We are confident in stating that a very considerable amount of this NHS money is NOT spent on GPs, hospital doctors, nurses and equipment to provide treatment to patients. A massive amount is wasted and spent on vast overheads by the autocratic, all-powerful, unaccountable and dictatorial NHS Commissioning Board, which has decided to call itself *NHS England*. Its self-importance and somewhat deceitful ostentatiousness is evident from its website. Created in March 2013, it appears as follows:
NHS England. 70 years OF THE NHS, 1948-2018.

Absolutely nowhere on the website does its legal name, NHS Commissioning Board, appear, which gives the impression that NHS England has been in operation for 70 years.

According to Full Fact, in 2017/18, NHS England received a sum of £122 billion. However, in its analyses, NHS England showed a sum of £109.3 billion, of which the Clinical Commissioning Groups received £73.6 billion. The rest – £35.7 billion – was kept by NHS England for what appears to be matters unrelated to improving unacceptable waiting lists.

Please note: NHS England is *not* the NHS in England. It is the biggest quango in the world, employing 6,500 staff in 50 locations to pretend to manage the affairs of the National Health Service in England.

The managers and politicians related to the NHS hold the following unanimous view:
'The reason for the shortcomings of the NHS are ageing population, expensive new techniques of diagnosis and the escalating cost of new drugs and treatment.'

Believe it or not, in 1979, a Royal Commission on the NHS stated, 'There are concerns that include an ageing population and the cost of technological developments.'

The solution, according to those running the NHS, is simple: more money.

We are the first to shout out about how the NHS management structure, which is run by the state from a sprawling, central, uncontrollable and unaccountable administration, is not fit for purpose and will never work, no matter how much money is put in this bottomless pit. This is the main reason why the NHS is not working.

Chapter Seven

Grapes of Wrath

The NHS is not working because its state-controlled management structure leads to monumental wastage of money. We beg you to please read the following:

The total private finance initiative debt to the NHS is over £300 billion for projects worth only £55 billion. This means that £245 billion has been wasted swelling the coffers of private companies.

Staff sickness absence costs £2.4 billion a year – £1 for every £40 of the total NHS budget. Forty-five thousand employees call in sick daily. NHS staff sickness is 2.5 times higher than in the private sector.

Ninety-eight NHS staff members get paid more than the UK Prime Minister. Over 600 quango chiefs are on six-figure salaries.

In 2015/16, the NHS spent an estimated £3.7 billion on agency costs (locum doctors and nurses).

The Robin Hood NHS steals money from taxpayers to offer free treatment to health tourists at a cost of over £1.8 billion a year.

In 2014, a year-long study by the professional body representing doctors found that the NHS wastes £2.3 billion a year on a range of procedures and processes that could be done better, cheaper or not at all.

The NHS handed over £750 million to EU countries for treatment of Britons abroad and claimed back just £50.3 million.

Primary care trust managers were paid £225 million in redundancy payments. Many moved the next day to the newly created CCGs.

Pharmaceutical companies have bought NHS officials tickets for sports matches and pop concerts to the tune of over £5 million and failed to declare £3.8 million on the public register. This practice of 'bribery' is not allowed and at the very least should be declared when it takes place.

The NHS has no system in place to avoid the wastage of £1 billion a year caused by the failure of patients to keep their appointments.

The NHS spends millions of pounds a year to provide translation services in 123 languages.

Would you believe it? This isn't fake news, or a misprint.

The NHS paid £1,322.52 for a 400gm tube of cortisone cream costing £1.90.

In May 2016, the NHS paid £1,579 for a 500ml tube of moisturiser costing £1.73.

One hospital paid £16.47 for a single pack of 12 rubber gloves that should have cost 35 pence.

Another splashed out £21.86 for one box of plasters costing £1.68.

The most damaging aspect of the mismanagement of the state-run monopoly is the abuse of sickness absence.

Private sector staff sickness absence =1.8%

Public sector   =2.9%

NHS   =4.4%

Statistics indicate that NHS staff absence due to sickness is 15 days per employee per year. This absence costs £2.4 billion a year. In other words, £1 for every £40 of the total NHS budget. The NHS is sick – metaphorically and literally.

NHS trusts have spent millions on external management consultants, which has led to a significant rise in inefficiency and, ultimately, worsening services. This was the conclusion of a study of 120 English trusts, which was carried out by academics at the University of Bristol and Warwick Business School. We have figures available for the year 2014, in which a sum of £640 million was spent on management consultants alone.

Figures from NHS annual reports for 2016/17 disclose managers at the 'struggling NHS CCGs' on rates equal to £200,000 a year, including five on more than £300,000 a year.

Examples:

Enfield CCG: Hired Mike Seitz at £34,000/month, paid for five months equal to an annual salary of £408,000.

North, East and West Devon: Paid Martin Shield £90,000 for three months equal to an annual rate of £360,000.

Surrey Downs CCG: Brought in Anthony Collins for £30,000 a month.

North Hampshire CCG: Paid Paul Sly at £310,000 for 11 months, plus £30,000 expenses.

All these people were hired by the 32 'struggling' 32 CCGs to put their affairs in order under the legal directions of NHS England – the biggest quango in the world – during 2016/17. The reason given was that 'their financial problems or quality of local services were so poor that they were deemed to be failing or at risk of failing to perform their basic functions'.

It appears that after spending all this money, 29 out of 32 CCGs are still struggling.

NHS bankruptcy is avoided on a daily basis by the state pouring in more and more money.

The breathtakingly negligent lack of financial control and accountability, with such colossal wastage of money, is one of the reasons WHY, the NHS is not working.

Chapter Eight

Ground control to Major Tom
Have you seen NHS Reform?
BALKANISED FIEFDOMS

The Mid Staffs Hospital's disaster man and the CEO of the NHS from 2008-2014, comrade (Sir) David Nicholson, cried the following words upon seeing the Health & Social Act 2012 and its proposed reforms, "These reforms are so huge that you can see them from outer space."

Jeremy Hunt, the health secretary from 2012 to July 2018, was in awe of David Nicholson and was in full agreement with the 2012 reforms. When Nicholson retired in 2014, Hunt heaped huge praise on him. As we mentioned earlier, NHS leadership takes its time to find out the truth, usually years after the event. The NHS took nine years to find out that 275,000 women were never sent appointments for breast cancer screening.

Andrew Lansley, who was the health secretary in 2012, later bitterly pointed out that he'd fallen victim to the failure of a bowel cancer-screening programme he'd proposed in 2010. It had still not been implemented by 2018.

You may remember that the constitution of the NHS was written in 2011, 63 years after its creation in 1948. You may ask why we are pointing out these NHS delays. Well, Jeremy Hunt, an admirer and advocate of the 2012 Act reforms, repented after four years and in May 2018 stated:

'The legislation has balkanised NHS into fiefdoms.'

Not having had the benefit of reading English at Oxford or teaching the language in Japan, as Mr Hunt did, we decided to humbly take advantage of a dictionary.

Balkanise:
To divide (a country or territory) into small, ineffectual states.
To divide (a region or body) into smaller, mutually hostile states or groups.

Fiefdom:
A territory or sphere of operation controlled by a particular person or group.
An area over which a person or organisation exerts authority or control.

We request that you please try and interpret what Mr Hunt means by his aforementioned fiefdoms statement.

At the end of this chapter, we will provide you with a list of the so-called white papers, green papers and other attempted reforms from 1950 to 2018.

A detailed study of these attempted changes would show that most of these so-called 'NHS reorganisations' were, in reality, half-baked and untested ideas based on the political ideology of the governments in power. A recent report by The King's Fund says that the 2012 Act failed to remove political influence from the NHS. Putting old vinegar into new bottles and declaring it vintage wine seems to have become the fashion.

The 1979 Royal Commission Report, which described the 'ageing population' and the cost of 'technological developments' as NHS problems is a good explanation for NHS failures today, as that was almost 40 years ago.

Labour created the concept of 'internal markets', only to later bitterly oppose it. The charade continued. In 2002, Alan Milburn (Labour) wanted to 'deliver the NHS'. Andrew Lansley replied by 'liberating the NHS' in 2010.

The net effect of these contradictory 'reorganisations' is Lansley's toxic legacy. Old PCTs (primary care trusts) with the same officials have now become 'conflict of interest ridden CCGs' headed by status ambitious, money loving but financially illiterate GPs.

The emergence of the centralist, all powerful, dictatorial and pretentious NHS Commissioning Board, posing as *NHS England* reminds one of George Orwell's note:
'One does not establish a dictatorship in order to safeguard a revolution, one makes a revolution to establish a dictatorship.'

We believe that the way the NHS is being run in England by NHS England (described by the British author and journalist Nicholas Timmins as the 'biggest quango in the world') poses a serious, existentialist threat to the NHS and is one of the reasons WHY it's not working.

Here is a list of white papers, green papers and attempted 'reorganisations' of the NHS:

1950: JS Collings Report the 'overall state of General Practice is bad & deteriorating'.

1951: One shilling (today's 5p) prescription charges.

1954: A review of the role of general practices encourages the formation of group practices. The Bradbeer committee report on the internal administration of hospitals.

1956: The Guillebaud committee enquiry into the cost of the NHS.

1959: Mental Health Act.

1962: Enoch Powell's hospital plan.

1966: Charter for General Practice.

1968: Seebohm Report. Kenneth Robinson's green paper. Ministry of Health merges with the Ministry of Social Security to form the Department of Health and Social Security.

1970: Crossman rewrites Robinson's proposals.

1972: Launch of the Cochrane report.

1973: NHS Reorganisation Act.

1976: Department of Health Resource Allocation Working Party Report.

1979: Royal Commission Report (Concerns include an ageing population and the cost of technological developments. The NHS is in no danger of collapse.)

1982: NHS reorganisation abolishes area health authorities.

1983: Mental Health Act 1983.

1985: Reflections on the management of the NHS by Professor Enthoven contributes to an NHS reform programme.

1986: Green paper on primary care.

1987: White paper 'promoting better health'.

1989: White paper 'working for patients' (NHS reforms).

1990: NHS reorganisation, the creation of the internal market and new GP contracts.

1991: The Patient's Charter.

1992: White paper: 'the health of the nation'; Tomlinson Report.

1994: NHS reorganisation.

1996: Three white papers released: 'choice and opportunity', 'primary care' and 'delivering the future and NHS'.

1997: White paper: 'The new NHS: modern, dependable.'

1998: A first-class service, quality in the new NHS. The Acheson Report on inequalities in health. Creation of NHS Direct.

1999: NHS reorganisation. GP fundholding abolished. White paper: 'our healthier nation'.

2000: The NHS Plan: a 10-year modernisation, investment and reform programme. Commission for healthcare improvement.

2001: The Health and Social Care Act 2001. The introduction of a hospital star-rating system.

2002: NHS reorganisation. The NHS 2002 Reform & Healthcare Professions Act. PCTs and SHAs created.

2003: NHS reorganisation: The Health & Social Care Act.

2003: New contracts for hospital consultants and GPs agreed.

2004: White paper: 'choosing health' published. NHS foundation trusts established. The Healthcare Commission takes over from Healthcare Improvement. Plans for GP practices in commissioning health care services.

2006: NHS reorganisation. SHAs reduced from 28 to 10 and PCTs from 303 to 152. White paper: 'our health, our care'.

2007: White paper: 'NHS autonomy & accountability'. Proposals for legislation.

2008: Health minister Lord Darzi's 10-year vision for the NHS: 'high quality care for all'.

2009: The NHS constitution published. Care Quality Commission created.

2009: David Nicholson, CEO of NHS England, announces efficiency savings in the NHS between £15 and £20 billion.

2010: Publication of Francis Enquiry report into Mid Staffordshire NHS Foundation Trust. Labour publishes white paper: 'building the National Care Service'. White paper: 'liberating the NHS'.

2012: Reorganisation of the NHS. 'Health & Social Care 2012' bill passed.

2013: New funding reforms for care and support (based on the Dilnot Commission in 2011). Robert Francis presents his final report.

2013, On 1 April, the new NHS comes into being with the shift of responsibilities based on the Health & Social Care Act 2012. In October, Simon Stevens is appointed CEO of NHS England.

2014: Autumn statement injects £2 billion into

NHS budget for 2015/16.

2016: On April 1, NHS Improvement is launched. Sustainability and transformation plans published.

2017: NHS England publishes: 'next steps on the five years forward view'.

2018: NHS 10 year plan.

Chapter Nine

There are more things in heaven and earth, Horatio,
Than are dreamt of in your philosophy

We have studied in great detail what NHS politicians, managers and civil servants have been trying to do since 1948. During all this time, no one has ever discovered that:

'You cannot run GP services, A&E units, hospitals and mental health services if you do not have enough doctors, nurses and equipment.'

It is impossible to comprehend why this simple and fundamental fact has eluded the thinking and planning of NHS politicians and managers for the last 70 years.

We can say unreservedly that the current model, with its catastrophic failings, may have managed to provide a reasonable service had it ensured there were a sufficient number of doctors to see patients promptly, as well as enough nurses and equipment.

NHS managers have been unable to comprehend two factors that have had a great impact on the way medical services are provided. The first is people's ability to gather information about their medical problems from internet search engines. Patients are becoming increasingly knowledgeable about their 'perceived' medical conditions. No longer is a GP able to tell the patient, 'I am afraid nothing can be done, you will have to live with it.'

GPs, in their determination to do the best for the patient, must refer them to a specialist. If they don't, the well-informed patient can ask, 'Why not'? This inevitably results in an ever-increasing number of GP referrals.

Hundreds of conditions for which nothing could be done in the past are now preventable, treatable, curable or manageable – each one being well beyond the capability of a GP and requiring the input of a relevant specialist. Conversely, it is the GP who is left to treat complex chronic problems, which are dealt with by the 'super specialist' and then referred back.

The second factor is the advancement in specialisation of every field of medicine and surgery. Only 15 years ago, an orthopaedic surgeon would deal with every problem related to matters requiring surgical intervention in 'joints and bones'. In the modern world, one specialist will deal only with problems relating to the lower back, another with the cervical spine. Different specialists deal with problems related to shoulders only, hips only, knees only and hands only. This applies to most specialities.

The running joke of the orthopaedic specialist is, 'In the future, I will be dealing only with the right hand or the right knee and my colleague with the left side.' The super specialisation in every field of medicine naturally requires more trained specialists.

The shortage of hospital doctors leads to waiting times of five to six months to see a specialist and six to 12 months to have a surgical procedure, as we have repeatedly pointed out.

Since 2012, the waiting list for treatment in NHS England has risen 47% faster than the population.

Incompetent NHS managers have been unable to understand these visible changes and trends and have therefore failed to take corrective action. They haven't grasped, as already mentioned, the urgent need to increase the number of doctors in order to keep up with the changing medical landscape.

The worst 'crime' of the NHS is allowing the reduction in the number of nurses. There are thousands (not hundreds) of unfilled nursing vacancies all over the UK, including the constituency of the PM, Mrs. May. An astonishing dossier of concerns raised by nurses about the impact of staffing levels, compiled from 18,000 nurse submissions and shared with the *Observer,* states, "Full staffing levels are becoming a 'rare event'; some emergency patients are being sent home as a result.

 Experienced nurses say they believe they are seeing the worst shortages in decades." Compiled by the Royal College of Nursing, the report adds, "We are operating with the worst levels in operating theatres. Patient care is severely compromised due to staffing levels."

As if these unacceptable and negligent reductions in the number of doctors and nurses weren't enough, the NHS has commenced a planned programme to reduce the number of hospitals. In 1987, the NHS had 299,000 beds; in 2017 the number of beds had been reduced to 142,000, with the largest drop occurring in overnight mental health and learning disability facilities. These fell by 72.1% and 96.4%, respectively. Official figures show that between 2010 and 2016, there was a reduction of 12,000 beds.

The NHS has 2.7 beds per 1000 population; France has 6.2/1000 and Germany has 8.2/1000.

The NHS has fewer CT scanners – 8 per million – compared to the EU average of 21.4 and fewer MRI scanners – 6.1 million – compared to the EU average of 15.4.

Add to this a shortage of surgeons and specialists in all fields, and the misery of the people requires no imagination to envisage.

With shortage of GPs, specialists, surgeons, nurses, equipment, hospital beds, is it any wonder WHY the NHS is not working?

Chapter Ten

We are the hollow men,
we are the stuffed men

'Ask not what I can do for the NHS,
ask what the NHS can do for me.'

Since 1990, the following 'honourable ladies and gentlemen' have held the position of Secretary of State for Health.

Name	From	To	Months	In office
W. Waldegrave	2.11.90	10.4.92	17	Conservative
V. Bottomley	10.4.92	5.7.95	38	Conservative
S. Dorrell	5.7.95	2.5.97	22	Conservative
F. Dobson	3.5.97	11.10.99	28	Labour
A. Milburn	11.10.99	13.6.03	44	Labour
J. Reid	13.6.03	6.5. 05	23	Labour
P. Hewitt	6.5.05	27.6.07	23	Labour
A. Johnson	28.6.07	5.6.09	23	Labour
A. Burnham	5.6.09	11.5.10	11	Labour
A. Lansey	11.5.10	4.9.12	28	Conservative/LD
J. Hunt	5.9.12	9.7.18	72	Conservative
M. Hancock	10.7.18	current		Conservative

William Waldegrave: In 1994, he told a House of Commons Select Committee the following: 'On occasion, parliament is lied to. Not only does parliament get lied to, parliament knows this and accepts this because lying is seen to be a necessary part of the political process.'

Virginia Bottomley: In April 1993, *The Independent* newspaper reported a speech by Bottomley to CBI, which proposed, 'To privatise the NHS, except that the NHS patients would still be treated free, the service should buy more care from private hospitals and health companies such as BUPA.'

After leaving her job, Bottomley was appointed as the non-executive director of BUPA. By coincidence, BUPA was awarded a contract to carry out 6000 procedures a year for NHS patients.

In the House of Lords, Bottomley enthused about the Health and Social Care Bill 2012. She said, 'I give this bill an unequivocal and extraordinarily warm welcome.' Her mouth watered at the prospect of private work and she joined a number of 'for profit' health-related companies, such as International Resources Group, Odgers Berndtson and AkzoNobel.

Mr Stephen Dorrell: After leaving his position, he accepted a job as an adviser with a private firm targeting a £1 billion NHS contract. This caused lots of media protest.

Mr Frank Dobson: He continued to live in a council flat whilst earning a six-figure ministerial salary and despite owning a large property in Yorkshire. He had no problem with paying £160 a week for accommodation worth £1000/week.

The ever-ambitious health secretary resigned to run for Mayor of London. Unfortunately, he lost.

Alan Milburn: As the Labour party's cheerleader for the NHS, just nine months after leaving his position as health secretary, between March and September 2004, Milburn joined Bridgepoint, a firm 'heavily involved in financing private health care firms'. After he joined, Bridgepoint's subsidiary won a £16 million NHS contract.

There was much protest in 2005, as patients were being sent 20 miles away to a private scanner owned by Alliance Medical of Bridgepoint and purchased for £90 million when Mr Milburn was working for the company. Meanwhile, the NHS scanner was considerably underused.

In May 2013, Mr Milburn joined PwC as chair of the Health Industry Board to 'help the company grow in the health market'. This was much to the annoyance of Labour party supporters.

In January 2015, A M Strategy, owned jointly by Milburn and his partner Ruth Briel, made more than £500,000. Accounts show the company had accumulated £1,357,131 in profit at that time. All the work related to consultancy for private health companies. In February 2018, Milburn joined Ribera Salud, a hospital management company owned by the US giant Centene Corporation.

Incidentally, Milburn's health minister, Lord Hutton of Furness, joined the board of Circle Holdings, a private health provider that had won NHS contracts worth £285 million.

John Reid: Born to Mary, a factory worker, and a postman called John, Reid joined the communist party in 1972 at the age of 25. As health secretary, he awarded a 23% rise to GPs and converted the 24/7 service to Monday- Friday, 8am - 6pm. No weekends. An advocate of private health care, in 2005 he announced that 'private healthcare would benefit the poor'. He enjoyed a free, three-day stay in a luxury lakeside hotel in Geneva, courtesy of the future war criminal, Bosnian politician Radovan Karadzic. In 2010, he was elevated to the House of Lords.

Patricia Hewitt: After being health secretary, Hewitt became a special consultant to one of the NHS's largest chemists, Alliance Boots. She joined the private equity company Cinven, which bought 25 private hospitals from BUPA. She was caught by the Channel 4 programme *Dispatches* offering to use her contacts for £3000 a day.

Alan Johnson: Reminding everyone that he used to be a postman, Johnson criticised breast cancer patient Debbie Hirst for wanting to buy the cancer drug, Avastin, which wasn't available to her on the NHS, using her own money. He claimed, 'This way lies the end of the founding principles of the NHS.' A political analyst accused him of 'complete failure to deliver on major threats to the NHS, no delivery for patients and no delivery for health professionals; he is the postman that hasn't delivered.'

Andy Burnham: His tenure of 11 months was too short to attract the attention of private health companies.

Andrew Lansley: In 2010, Lansley accepted a donation of £21,000 for his private office from Caroline Nash, the wife of John Nash, who was the chairman of Care UK. At that time, Care UK was one of the largest private companies with NHS contracts.

The person responsible for introducing the 2012 Health & Social Care Act, Lansley resigned in September 2012 after the BMA's unprecedented vote of no confidence in him a few months earlier. He was told that he 'had misled both the public and the profession with respect to the detail and consequences of the Health & Social Care Act.'

The BMA added: 'How can we trust this man? It is clear that we have a health secretary who is ideologically bound, thinks he knows best, is disingenuous and sticks fingers in his ears.'

He now sits in the House of Lords and does advisory work for several private companies, including Roche, a pharmaceutical company at the centre of a row over the prices it charges the NHS, and the private equity firm Blackstone regarding investments in the health sector. He also lends his expertise to corporate clients on innovation in the health sector.

It is with regret that we note he has developed

bowel cancer. Paradoxically, he blames this on the NHS. In 2010, he claims to have introduced a programme called 'Bowel Scope' for men over 55. In 2018, it is still not in operation, which is typical of NHS management. We wish him the best for a full recovery.

Jeremy Hunt: His exploits as health secretary could easily be the subject of a bestselling book. He was the first health secretary in 48 years to provoke a junior doctors' strike and the longest serving, since 1990. He seems to have developed an expertise for forgetting, hence one of his nicknames, 'The Forgetful Jeremy'.

Between 2015 and 2016, Hunt forgot to attend all seven gatherings of the Department of Health board. All these meetings took place against the backdrop of the junior doctors' strike.

In 2018, he apologised to the British public for the A&E fiasco, which resulted in the cancellation of thousands of surgical procedures. He called it unacceptable.

Hunt had forgotten that he'd made a similar statement in 2013 about the same situation and promised that this kind of A&E crisis would not happen again. He allocated £250 million to the cause. Hunt is rather fond of using the word unacceptable when talking about each NHS public failing, but, of course, after using it he soon forgets.

In 2009, he accepted that he had 'forgotten' he was in breach of the rules of the House in making a claim for utilities and other services on his Farnham home in the period during which it was still his main residence. He repaid the sum claimed in full.

In 2012, he had a lapse in memory and received dividends from his company Hotcourses in the form of property, which was leased back to the company. The dividend in specie was paid just before a 10% rise in dividend tax, and he was not required to pay stamp duty on the property. According to *The Daily Telegraph*, this forgetfulness reduced his tax bill by £100,000.

Hunt did remember to set up a company, Mare Pond Properties, to purchase seven luxury flats with his wife Lucia Guo. He was accused of being in breach of the Companies Act on two accounts: he forgot that he should have declared to Companies House that he was the person 'with significant control' and the second person in the transaction with his wife. This is a criminal offence, punishable by a fine or up to two years imprisonment. His memory came back and he rectified the situation six months later.

He also forgot to disclose 50% of his interest of shareholding in Mare Pond Properties with the Register of Members' Financial Interests. Fortunately, five months later he remembered to do so.

As the Health Secretary, he said that homeopathy had no place in modern medicine. He then forgot this and promised to 'support NHS funding for it, if recommended by a doctor'. He also forgot that his company Hotcourses sold 'homeopathic medicine courses'.

He forgot about the time limit on termination of pregnancy in England and thought it best at no more than 12 weeks.

He forgot that he had said in an interview with *Health Service Journal* in 2014 that he wanted to remain as health secretary until 2017, continuing in office until July 2018.

He forgot his great enthusiasm for the Lansley 2012 Act and, in 2018, stated, 'The legislation has balkanised NHS into Fiefdoms.' He was appointed as Foreign secretary on 10th July and Matt Hancock took his place.

In August 2018, the ever-forgetful Jeremy, now Foreign Secretary, on his visit to China, forgot that his wife is Chinese and introduced her as 'Japanese'.

Matt Hancock was appointed the new health secretary on 10th July 2018 and proceeded to show his ignorance by joining Babylon and declaring "My GP is through the NHS on Babylon Health, it's brilliant".

This has forced us to delay the publication of this

book and add a special chapter on the subject, chapter 17.

In 2015, he is renowned to have chartered a private jet (on taxpayers' expense) as the Energy minister from Aberdeen to London, when it is reported that on that day there were available 16 scheduled flights to four London airports.

The Independent newspaper announced sensationally in July 2018 and we quote, exactly as it appeared:
"Mr. Hancock received £32,000 in donations from chair of think tank that wants NHS 'abolished'".

In 2014, as minister for energy and a strong advocate of fracking, he was interviewed on Radio 4's Today programme, rejecting the suggestion that fracking was unpopular. When challenged he was unable to name a single village that supported it.

He was pleased to accept a donation from Disciple Media Ltd. to create for him a personal app. The narcissist Mr. Matt Hancock named it, yes you have guessed it right, Matt Hancock.

Labour party was not pleased, when Mr. Hancock declared them as "a party full of queers", only to apologise and withdraw the tweet.

Looking at the records of several of these health secretaries, it becomes clear that many wanted to make a 'buck or two' by taking direct or indirect advantage of their positions. It is our view that with their qualifications and business sector experience, many would have struggled to secure even a job interview in a large PLC company.

Their personal character, their greed for power and money, especially after leaving their parliament job, speaks for itself. While claiming to be guardians and saviours of the NHS from private company encroachment, several took jobs from the very same private companies. Many are now sitting in the House of Lords.

(Sir) David Nicholson was the CEO of the NHS from 2006-2014. From the age of 22 until the age of 28, he was also a member of the UK's communist party (1977-1983). He was no ordinary revolutionary and belonged to the 'tankie wing' of the party, which backed the Kremlin using military action to crush the dissident uprising.

Being a member of the communist party for six years and knowing that Stalin had executed more than a million of his own people would automatically exclude him from holding high office in any commercial organisation. This would not be on account of his views, but rather the undeniable feebleness of his intellect and his support of a tyrannical, autocratic regime. At one point his idol was the Soviet dictator, Leonid Brezhnev (1964-83).

Before his appointment as the Chief Executive of the NHS, for two years David Nicolson was the man in charge of the notorious mismanagement of Stafford Hospital.

He retired in 2014 with a pension pot of £2 million for services rendered to the NHS.

Jeremy Hunt, who was the health secretary at the time of writing this book, was full of praise for this man, saying, 'Sir David Nicholson made the NHS better.'

This praise was effectively for the man responsible for the Mid Staffordshire NHS Foundation Trust's greatest scandal, where, 'Over 1200 patients died. Patients were left lying in their own urine and excrement, forced to drink water from vases and given wrong medication.' (Francis report)

In Sept 2011, Nicholson claimed expenses of over £50,000 a year on top of a basic salary of £200,000 and benefits of £37,600 at a time when he was claiming the NHS was short of money.

NHS appointments for key managerial jobs are there for taking. In 2007, builder Jon Andrews faked his CV and was made chairman of the NHS Torbay Care Trust. In 2015, he beat 117 others to become chairman of the Royal Cornwall NHS Trust.

(We have been unable to find how many of the applicants were from the building trade.)

With such recruitment policies of the NHS, it is of no surprise to learn that the disgraced NHS 'boss', who at 63 was dubbed the 'man with no shame', has been rehired by NHS Improvement at Worcestershire NHS Trust.

Simon Stevens, who was associated with the American company UnitedHealth Group from 2004–2014 as vice president and CEO, is the new CEO of *NHS England*. His duties in the UnitedHealth Group included lobbying for the NHS and other European health services to be included in TTIP (Transatlantic Trade and Investment Partnership), which would allow international companies to compete for NHS services by the private sector.

After four years in office, no improvement in the NHS is visible. His experience in a US company, with its core business of health insurance, seems incompatible with the NHS's ethos.
Abraham Maslow said, 'If all you have is a hammer, everything looks like a nail.' Stevens' US health insurance hammer experience has the NHS for nails.

Greedy past and present NHS leaders, with no experience of how universal healthcare systems work, no business acumen, no vision, no accountability and no fear of financial deficits, have created a Molotov cocktail that explains WHY the NHS is NOT working.

How can the NHS be changed to Put Patients First

Chapter Eleven

If you don't know where you are going,
any road will take you there

We hope that by now you will agree that the NHS is a broken system. Please don't take our word for it. A report in 2018 by the Institute for Fiscal Studies said, 'Health spending must increase from £154 billion to £249 in future, just to maintain the present level of service.' Analysts are of the view that the NHS needs £2000 a year in tax from every household just to stay afloat. The IFS emphasised that, 'the resources needed far outstrip any tax pledges made'.

A penny on all main rates of income tax would raise £6 billion; a penny on VAT would raise £6 billion, a penny on each of the employee, self-employed and employer's National Insurance contributions would raise £10 billion. With these fairly aggressive tax rises, the total amount is just £22 billion.

And, if you consider the massive amounts the NHS needs now and, in the future, with horrendous waiting times for patients, the only conclusion has to be that the NHS must change. Putting more and more cash into this bottomless pit could bankrupt the economy but would do nothing to alter this pathetic dinosaur.

We have a solution, a new model for the NHS that would provide a health service to UK residents similar to the ones in France, Germany, the Netherlands and most European countries, while mirroring their budgetary disciplines.

Before we describe in detail our proposed NHS model, which would help eliminate most problems, we need to examine the current financial arrangements.

'NHS privatisation' must be one of the most loathed and feared terms amongst the British public and the most loved by politicians of all political parties.

Labour politicians, after commenting on hurricanes, earthquakes, floods and political turmoil, conclude by saying, 'We will safeguard our NHS from the Conservative party's privatisation plan.' The Conservatives, after speeches on hurricanes, earthquakes, floods and political turmoil, will add, 'Unlike the Labour party, the NHS is safe in our hands and we have no intention to privatise it.'

What does the privatisation of the NHS mean? Does it mean that our free NHS services will be replaced by everyone 'buying' GP and specialist consultations, medical investigations, surgical procedures and ambulance calls? Or does it mean that all medical and care services would be provided by 'for profit companies'?

Does the rumour that Simon 'US Private Health Insurance' Stevens, CEO of NHS England, wants to 'privatise' the NHS and turn into the pitiful US health care model have any substance?

Our research into the definition of 'privatisation' is as follows:
'A part of the NHS appears to be privatised when any service is 'contracted' to a 'for profit company' instead of NHS employees, or when people pay for an NHS service. The so-called 'privatisation' involves three distinct types of health-related services:

CLINICAL:
1. This involves contracting services provided by NHS hospital doctors to private hospitals and GP services to the private companies. We have dealt in detail with treatment of patients in private hospitals by fully employed, six-figure salaried NHS doctors in order to make fat profits for private hospitals, private health insurance companies and themselves.

We have devoted a special and additional chapter to the emergence of private companies which offer next day GP appointments.

We have excellent recommendations to eliminate both of the above practices.

2. NHS Dentistry was 'privatised' in 1951, three years after the creation of the NHS. Unlike the generous exemptions that the NHS gives to the over 65s and unemployed, etc., everyone over the age of 18 must pay for their dental work. Here's

a rundown of the cost of NHS dental services, which are not cheap, as of April 2018:
Band one: £21.60; band two: £59.10; band three: £256.50.

3. The NHS charge for an eye test is £21.31, and if the person wants an eye test at home due to a physical handicap, for instance, it's £37.56 (April 2018).

4. A prescription charge is £8.80 per item (April 2018).

5. Miscellaneous NHS charges: Surgical brassiere: £28.85, abdominal support: £43.60, spinal support: £43.60, stock wig: £71.25, partial human hair wig: £188.70 and a full human hair wig: £275.95.

6. Hearing Aids: This industry was 'privatised' decades ago. Millions of people now pay for their aids because of substandard and bulky free NHS aids.

SEMI-CLINICAL:
Community and social-related services, which may require NHS trained nurses and the background support of GPs.

Details of private company contracts to non-NHS providers, April 2010 to April 2015:
86% pharmacy services
83% patient transport services
76% diagnostic services

69% GP/out-of-hour services
45% community health services
25% mental health services

In the year 2016/17, 386 contracts (almost 70%) – worth £3.1 billion – went to the private sector.

Long Term Care of the Elderly: This became an increasing problem more than 25 years ago. Local councils with small residential homes found that they didn't have the expertise to run such homes. The Independent Residential & Nursing Care Home sector was thus born.

Councils or the NHS now provide less than 10% of this type of social care. In other words, more than 90% of all social care relating to residential and nursing care of the elderly has been 'privatised'. This happened years ago, with the full approval of both the Labour and Conservative parties in power.

And 83% of all providers are 'for profit companies', with the others being charities and voluntary organisations.

Over the years, this sector has grown massively. The total available capacity of beds in all non-NHS care homes is 454,000 beds in 11,293 homes. It's worth noting that NHS hospitals had just 142,568 beds in 2016–17. Therefore, the non-NHS care home sector has 3.18 times more beds than all the NHS hospitals. The care home sector is worth £15.9 billion a year.

On average, 41% of residents are self-funded and pay for their care. There is a vigorous method of assessment on the ability to pay. It is worth noting that the 'means testing' mechanism has been in place for over 25 years, unnoticed by those who are fiercely opposed to this concept.

It's also interesting to document that 59% of people in non-NHS care home beds are funded by the state. During the huge transfer of care from the state to the independent and private sector, the process of commissioning did not exist. The independent residential and nursing home model is an example of the state sharing the financial burden of care with 'for profit' providers and individuals. This totally contradicts the NHS motto 'free for all, equal for all'. It also establishes 'means testing' before free entitlement to a service. All care is neither free for all nor equal for all.

Domiciliary Care of the Elderly:
According to the figures available to us, there were 8,800 domiciliary care services registered with CQC in Sept 2016. These care providers had around 505,000 jobs between them. About 96% of these were in the independent sector.

It appears that up to 673,000 people are receiving domiciliary care in England. The figure available for direct expenditure on domiciliary care for 2014/15 was £3.3 billion, with local authorities contributing £2.6 billion, self-funders £623 million and with the total expenditure on direct payment amounting to £1.4 billion.

NON-CLINICAL:
These include general administration services, hospital building maintenance, catering, laundry cleaning and IT, etc. (We can't help telling you that one hospital had to pay £350 to change a light bulb under the contract conditions of the notorious Private Finance Initiative (PFI).)

A recent report is damning of NHS England for outsourcing to its favourite private company, Capita. The National Audit Office (we are great fans of this organisation) has said that the £330 million seven-year contract is a 'textbook example of how to set up an outsourcing contract to fail'. Capita has lost £125 million in the first two years and both parties seem to be at war with each other.

We hope that we have adequately explained what the 'privatisation' of the NHS means. We have explained the difference between people paying for NHS services (dentistry, prescriptions, eye tests, hearing aids, etc.) and the NHS services that have been contracted to 'for profit companies'.

We have provided details of the long-term care of the elderly in nursing and residential homes and domiciliary care, which now is a massive sector in its own right. The salient features of this kind of care are:

All 'care' is neither 'free for all, nor equal for all'.

The majority of domiciliary care and the running of residential and nursing homes have for many years been carried out privately by 'for-profit companies'. The state pays these companies to provide the care. The state also makes every effort to make individuals pay for their care, if they are able to afford it. This is decided through a means test.

The NHS uses large 'for profit companies' based in the US and 'offshore tax havens' to supply non-clinical and semi-clinical services.

The NHS and the Department of Health do not have a fixed and consistent policy on who pays, who does not, what services an individual would pay for and what are free. Prescription and eye test charges are free for men above the age of 65 and for women above 60. But everyone must pay the fairly expensive dentistry charges.

GP consultations, A&E visits and all hospital services are free, but people must pay for prescriptions, eye tests, surgical brassieres, abdominal supports, spinal supports, stock wigs, partial human hair wigs and fully bespoke human hair wigs, etc.

The state aggressively assesses who can pay for their private care in a nursing home by means testing and, as already stated, 41% of people do have to cover this themselves. And yet individuals continue to occupy beds in hospitals with no clinical need to do so due to social reasons, which causes havoc in the entire NHS hospital system. The NHS makes no demand to these people to pay for immediate alternate accommodation.

I hope you have been able to judge for yourself the nightmarish 'public money charging' model of the NHS, where incompetence and inaction meet inconsistency.

How does this all fit in with the original philosophy of the then minister of health, Aneurin Bevin? On July 5th 1948, he said,
'The NHS is based on the principles:
1. *That it meet the needs of everyone.*
2. *That it be free at the point of delivery.*
3. *That it be based on clinical needs, not the ability to pay.*'

Poor Mr Bevin ... obviously he had no clever adviser to correct his grammar, or to tell him that out of his main three principals number two and three are exactly the same. Number one called for the 'NHS to meet the needs of everyone', and these needs are in goal three under 'clinical needs'.

According to NHS Choices, these three principles have guided the development of the NHS for the past 70 years and remain at its core.

NHS Choices goes on to explain that it took the NHS 63 years to publish its constitution in 2011, which has seven principles. These contain improved grammar but seem to have been written by a prize-winning novelist, as none of them have come close to reality since 1948 and, for that matter, 2011, including Bevin's announcement that the service would be free at the point of delivery.

The thousands of wealthy women from around the world who enjoy 'free delivery of babies' in NHS hospitals (excuse the pun), and the hundreds of thousands of rich people who fly daily to the UK to have FREE treatment would testify to the generosity and philanthropy of Bevin's philosophy. (The annual cost of health tourism is £1.8 billion.) The NHS's charity knows no bounds; it provides free translation services in 123 languages, so that UK taxpayers are able to provide free medical services to those with enough money to fly here but not enough English language skills.

Excluding the talented, dedicated and long-suffering doctors and nurses, we can safely say that the NHS is being run for the benefit of its 1.7 million employees, six-figure salaried quango managers and ever-ready, greedy management consultants. The patients seem to be a bit of a nuisance and ungrateful for Mr Bevin's free treatment.

The NHS aspires to put patients at the heart of everything it does, as long as they can learn and accept that The National Health Service is now the 'waiting health service'.

The NHS is commercially insolvent with a budget of £147.5 billion in 2017/18 (this is more than the GDP of 140 countries out of 192).

The main message of this book continues to be:

You have no idea of the physical pain people go through as they wait for months to be seen or have an operation. You have no idea of the anguish people with mental health problems go through as they wait six to 12 months to see someone, often while feeling suicidal. You have no idea how it feels not to be able to get an appointment to see a GP for weeks at a time when your child is ill. You have no idea how it feels to lie on a trolley in A&E for hours amongst dozens of people, as if it was a war zone.

The NHS has no tangible goals for an easy and early access to its services, except that it be free at the point of delivery. The NHS has no tangible goals to identify why some services are free, while others, similar or dissimilar, cost money. The NHS has not set goals to find out why rules were established to offer contracts to 'for profit tax havens/US companies' when the legal costs and other expenditures related to the contracting process sometimes cost more than the amount of money saved.

The NHS has never set goals to find out what did it cost to create the so-called (sham) internal markets and more importantly, how much does it cost to run it. The NHS has never set goals to find out why millions of pounds are being spent on creating giant administration quangos just to distribute money to hospitals, GPs and the community.

The NHS has never bothered to set goals to find out what were the evidence-based facts behind the disastrous 2012 Act before implementation.

The NHS is like Alice in Wonderland; it doesn't know where it is going, any road will take it there, and it is going nowhere.

Chapter Twelve

A Farewell to Arms

Since 1948, when the NHS was born, almost everything has changed in the world we live in. So many life and lifestyle transformations have occurred: computers, cheap holiday travel, the fall of communism, the EU, satellites, colour TVs, mobile phones and the invention of the internet, to mention but a few.

The only things that have not changed are the laws of nature and the waiting lists of the NHS.

You will agree that with the evidence provided, an NHS run by people with neither ability nor vision, who are trying to provide health services to 66.5 million people through 1.7 million employees, is a disaster. The chronic shortage of funds due to gross mismanagement leads to constant demand for more money.

It's time to say goodbye to the 70-year-old baby, which is still playing with its toys and demanding more candy.

We have a detailed alternative plan that we are confident will work. The proposed model would be called **NHS for us** with the following goals:

General Practice: Same-day appointments available with a maximum wait of one to two days. We have a short-term plan to provide after hours and weekend cover.

Hospital Specialists: A one-week waiting time to see any specialist, a maximum of two.

Surgery: A maximum waiting period of two weeks.

A&E: A maximum waiting time of one hour, two if there were unexpected emergencies.

Ambulances: A waiting time of 10 to 15 minutes.

MRI & CT Scans: One week.

Finances: The agreed annual budget would be adhered to. The existing NHS practice of daily insolvency would be abolished.

Principal of Universal Health Care: Access to all medical services, without the ability to afford, would be maintained.

To the people in the UK, and those running the NHS, the above would be utopia, a utopia that is impossible to achieve. However, please be assured that these health care arrangements are normal practice in France, Germany, the Netherlands and several other of the EU countries where Universal Healthcare is in place.

Our proposed **NHS for us** model, at this stage, is applicable to England only.

The major change would involve decentralisation of the existing NHS management structure.

In spite of the ruthless closure of hospitals and

the reduction of beds from 299,000 in 1987 to 142,000 in 2017, the nucleus of all non-GP health provision is the 150 or so main hospitals in England. These hospitals are geographically placed to be able to cover a catchment area of 275,000 to 350,000 people and serve the entire population of England. Larger hospitals may provide services to a greater number of people and may have more advanced and specialised facilities to treat patients from neighbouring hospitals.

Each NHS hospital is a 'centre of excellence' and has been so throughout the history of the NHS.

Our new model '**NHS for us**' is based on devolving all the services controlled by *NHS England* to each hospital, which would become a *Local NHS Centre*. Thus, there would be a transfer from one massive, super quango *NHS England* to 150 or so regional hospitals, that we have named *Local NHS Centres*.

The undeniable fact is that these hospitals have already been providing specialist services to their local community, including endocrinology, cardiology, ear, nose and throat, gynaecology, geriatrics, gastro enterology, haematology, nephrology, neurology, obstetrics, oncology, ophthalmology, orthopaedics, paediatrics, pathology, rheumatology, radiology, radiotherapy and respiratory. They have also been providing surgical procedures for a vast variety of diseases, and A&E and diagnostic facilities, including blood tests, scans and x-rays.

Without exception, these hospitals have doctors, nurses and support technicians that are unmatched in any such institution in the world and offer a truly outstanding service. Reminder, these hospitals in new model **NHS for us,** would be called *Local NHS Centres.*

Each *Local NHS Centre* would be registered as a charity with the Charity Commission. Local captains of business and industry would be invited to become trustees, and each trustee would be expected to provide expertise in various areas of finance and management. They would establish an independent management structure to provide every local clinical requirement, including GP and community services.

Local NHS Centres would operate independently. They would review existing loans, staffing levels and service agreements and, where feasible, negotiate new contracts. One of the major changes would be the provision of GP services to the local community, thus reversing the existing dynamics of the NHS management structure.

Each *Local NHS Centre* would work in cooperation with neighbouring units and synergise their services rather than competing. Their main relationship with central government would be to do with funding (this will be discussed later on in the book).

The benefits of decentralisation and devolution of powers and administration from *NHS England* to regional and local hospitals, acting as *Local NHS Centres* are immense. The massive, Soviet-style sprawling infrastructure, employing an enormous workforce with useless quangos at the cost of millions would be abolished. The *Local NHS Centres* would give ownership of medical service provision to the local community, which would work together and take pride in excelling through participation.

The dictatorial and faceless ignorant managers, supported by fat cat and equally ignorant consultants ruling from taxpayer-funded opulent office buildings situated hundreds of miles away, would disappear. These would be replaced by local people, caring for local communities and allocating every penny to having more doctors, more nurses, more GPs, more equipment and at the same time eliminating colossal money wastage through incompetence, ignorance and negligence.

The latest NHS spending scandal revealed by *The Times* in May 2018 is shocking (even though we have given examples of similar NHS wastage before).

The NHS paid:
£2,600 for basic sleeping pills that can cost the equivalent of £1 in US supermarkets.

£3,200 for arthritis painkillers that have cost less

than £1 per pack.

£45 for one tablet for an ulcer medicine, which can cost 13p.

This heart breaking waste of taxpayers' money will NEVER occur when local hospitals, with local trustees and local financial experts acting for *Local NHS Centres*, are in control.

The *Local NHS Centres* would use local businesses and companies to provide competitive services and improve the local economy. They will not use 'for profit companies' based in the United States or tax havens that improve shareholders' profits. The *Local NHS Centres* would revive small local satellite hospitals, which provide invaluable services to the local community against the contemptuous centralisation policies of the last CEO of the NHS, comrade (Sir) David Nicolson.

You may remember the *failed* 'NHS, IT Grand Plan,' which cost British taxpayers £12 billion. The *Local NHS Centres* would not need to produce complex systems for serving the entire UK population of 66.5 million people.

Fiascos such as failing to realise for nine years that 475,000 women hadn't been sent breast screening appointments, which caused innumerable premature deaths, would no longer happen.

Every *Local NHS Centre* would produce its own

cost-effective and efficient systems to cater to the needs of a small local community. The cold, faceless, remote, bulky services of the NHS would become local, precise, warm and personalised.

All services of the NHS Commissioning Board, posing as *NHS England* and propped up by its sycophantic, useless quangos, which cost taxpayers hundreds of millions to exist, would be devolved to the local communities and dismantled for good.

The charade of creating internal markets to 'purchase services' that the hospitals have been providing for years, which works on the principal of robbing Peter to pay Paul, would come to an end. The people being paid more than our PM to run an insolvent NHS, which makes people to wait for months in misery and anguish, would find out that the private sector gives no such handouts.

One of the priorities of *Local NHS Centres* would be to challenge, negotiate and terminate where possible, the toxic loans of Private Finance Initiative and refuse to pay £350 for changing an electric bulb (as we discovered in one case).

The creation of *Local NHS Centres* would transform the old, unworkable NHS to the new model, **'NHS for us'** 'of the local People, by the local People, for the local People.'

Chapter Thirteen

A Tale of Two Cities
Let there be an age of wisdom,
it was an era of foolishness

In order to understand better, the proposed new NHS model **NHS for us,** based on *Local NHS Centres* let us find out how the NHS works financially. Historically, chancellors of the exchequer have given money to the NHS from what they thought the country could afford, without ever finding what amount was really required.

Once the amount was decided, the state had to find how to distribute the money to each hospital and GP, plus other services, including community services, drugs and medicines, etc.

On 1st April 2013, it was decided that PCTs should be abolished and replaced with 'Clinical Commissioning Groups'. The process of allocating money from 1st April to present is that the treasury provides funds to the various devolved regions: Scotland, Wales, Northern Ireland and the all-powerful, super-quango, NHS Commissioning Board, which is posing as NHS England.

NHS England then makes decisions to distribute money as it deems fit, and keeps the rest itself to administer the massive, Soviet-style management structure and quangos it created.

Now, please have a look at the process of distributing money by the *NHS England,* with the following players:
Clinical commissioning groups, commissioning support units , lead provider framework.

Not content with the above arrangements, NHS England is now creating 44 'sustainability and transformation partnerships' to 'remove the division between buyers and sellers' in the NHS.

The concept of internal markets in the NHS as purchaser/ provider, and the creation of commissioning to deliver it, is so intellectually juvenile and practically unimplementable that on close examination, one does not know whether to laugh or cry over the shambles it has managed to create.

Traditionally, every hospital in England provides a comprehensive range of inpatient, outpatient, emergency and diagnostic services and covers, on average, a population of 275,000 to 350,000. This has not changed for decades.

In spite of extensive research, we have been unable to find out how *NHS England* through its maze of quangos is going to 'purchase' a service that the hospital is already providing. Would it be specialist consultations? Surgical procedures? Diagnostic investigation? Where would this be 'purchased' from? A neighbouring NHS hospital, situated miles away, because it is cheaper?

The unbelievable nonsense is that the *NHS England* from the funds provided by the government, is now pretending to 'purchase' services from NHS-funded hospitals that they are already providing. This typically NHS deceitful process is called 'commissioning'.

To give an example, the local community the hospital serves may require 500 cataract operations. *NHS England,* through the clinical commissioning group and other quangos may decide that only 400 operations can be 'purchased' this year. The other 100 people requiring this vital procedure will have to live with their near blindness for the next 12 months. This complex process is called 'commissioning'! In good old communist times, this used to be called 'rationing' and everyone living in the Soviet Union and its satellites, at the time, understood it.

With the clinical commissioning task done, now all they have to do is 'purchase other services'. Why allow the present system to continue when a tax haven or US-based company may do a better job and make a good profit for the owners? Never mind if the legal and financial cost of the contract exceeds any savings.

Imagine now, please, that the clever *NHS England* has decided to 'commission and buy' some surgical procedures and consultations from private hospitals. These everyday procedures will now be performed by the NHS's fully employed consultants within the private hospital sector, making a fat profit for the private hospital owners, the private health insurance companies and the NHS consultants themselves – all paid for by the taxpayers.

We have already established that in reality, the private hospital sector only exists because of free patronage by the NHS and its specialist doctors and surgeons. (Please do refer to Chapter Two, where the sham existence of the private hospital sector is exposed.)

This so-called 'commissioning' of a consultation, surgical procedure or diagnostic test from a private hospital by the *NHS England* is so outrageously scandalous and unethical, that it can be 'seen from the outer space', as the comrade, David Nicolson, the outgoing CEO of NHS England (2008–14), predicted upon the introduction of the 2012 Act.

Going back to the financial model of '**NHS for us,** based on *Local NHS Centres*, it is simple and in keeping with the globally applicable principals of running an enterprise. It would involve finding out about the true and accurate operational cost for eliminating, once and for all, constant funding deficits and abolishing unacceptable waiting lists.

Amazingly, no one in the NHS has ever tried to find out the following:
1. The additional number of GPs, hospital doctors

and nurses required to produce a zero-waiting list in all clinical-related services.

2. The additional diagnostic equipment required to produce a zero-waiting list: MRI scanners, CT scanners, radiotherapy and path lab equipment, etc.

3. The additional staff required to service the new equipment.

4. The number of beds that can be contracted out to local nursing homes or similar so patients who are occupying beds due to non-medical reasons can be discharged from wards.

5. Other deficiencies in funding.

Now, if you could add up the above five, this would give the true cost of running the NHS to the same standards as, say, the French, the Germans or the Dutch.

If you remember, in the budget of Nov 2017, the total revenue of the UK from all taxes was declared to be £769 billion, of which the money allocated to the NHS was £147.5 billion (£147,500,000,000), representing approximately 20% of the total UK tax revenue.

We'd like to know the total funds requirement of the NHS annually so that it is never short of money and has enough doctors, nurses and equipment to provide a prompt access to all its services to the patients. Does the NHS need £200 billion a year, £250 billion a year to achieve this desirable result?

The NHS is unable to answer this vital question. How can you operate an organisation like NHS, if you don't know the real annual funding requirements?

In summary, the complex, bureaucratic, market-style NHS infrastructure we have today would be dismantled in order to allocate funds directly to each regional hospital *Local NHS Centre* which would be acting as a charity (the infrastructure of which has already been explained in chapter 12).

Funding to each *Local NHS Centre* would be based on the principal of zero-waiting lists for every service through the recruitment of more GPs, specialists and consultants and the purchase of more equipment and staff to run it.

NHS for us would stop the nonsense of depriving people of vital services while financially illiterate and conflict of interest-ridden clinical commissioning groups and their master, *NHS England,* pretend to 'purchase' services from the same NHS hospital. The deceitful and shameful practice of 'buying' the clinical services from private hospitals, through NHS fully employed specialists, would be abolished.

Our recommended model of the NHS may appear to be somewhat 'revolutionary', but nothing could be simpler or make more sense. Our first call is for politicians to be straight with the British public and to stop playing silly games. The government in power has to state the accurate and real amount required to run a health service without communist-style rationing and the insufferable misery of those waiting to access services.

What would it cost to have enough GPs, hospital doctors and diagnostic equipment so that no one had to wait to access any of the services? It's time to tell the truth and announce whether the UK government is able to deliver the same service as other European countries.

If the government can't afford it, then it should come clean and say loud and clear, 'We do not have enough money to run the NHS as it is being run now.' It is time to stop the charade of cheating people through unproven reforms and wasting vulgar amounts of money on breathtakingly incompetent and negligent administration.

We are absolutely confident that the recommended model of **NHS for us** would deliver the double benefits of zero waiting lists and zero financial deficit by paying the required funds directly to each *Local NHS Centre*. This would result in the cessation of NHS England and all its quangos.

How would the incestuously interwoven vested interests of multibillion-pound industries, involving private health insurance companies, private hospitals and the people in *NHS England* with its quangos earning vast sums of money, react to this proposal? How would the US-based private companies and enterprises situated in tax havens, which are vying to make big profits from the NHS, respond? They would do everything in their power to stop it, wouldn't they?

NHS for us operating from local hospitals as *Local NHS Centres*, of the local People, by the local People, for the local People, is the only way forward.

Chapter Fourteen

Corridors of Power

We have investigated the NHS waiting list phenomenon going back as far as the 1970s. It appears that the NHS has *always* had a waiting list, which has continued to lengthen.

We discovered that the NHS waiting list is like a dog following its tail and going round and round. The dog will never catch its tail, leading to the huge suffering of those involved and a chronic collapse of NHS services.

We analysed hospital waiting lists. It became clear that the number of patients seen by every consultant in all specialities, and the number of elective surgical procedures in all specialities, in any given period, is less than what is required, based on the number of GP referrals.

The consequence of seeing fewer patients in each speciality by each specialist in one given week, in relation to the number actually required, leads to an increasing number of people waiting for a longer period. Here is a hypothetical but true situation, which doesn't divulge true numbers.

Let us assume that the number of patients referred by their GPs to a specialist is, on average, 20 per week. We know that this number is never achieved (otherwise there would be no waiting lists). Let us assume again that the number of patients actually seen by the specialist per week is 12, and it is impossible for them to see any more. This would leave eight patients waiting to be seen this week. There is every reason to believe that this pattern would be repeated every week, with the possibility of more referrals being required.

Under these circumstances, every consultant would have at least 416 patients on their waiting list at the end of one year, and so on.

The delay in consultations by specialists, it appears, can only be due to the fact that the number of specialists available to see the number of patients referred by their GPs is not enough. The same is applicable for surgical procedures.

Logically, the NHS would have an increasing number of people waiting to be seen in every speciality and in every passing week.

It is a mystery how the NHS manages to cope with the above mathematical calculation. With every research tool at our disposal, we have not been able to solve this riddle. How does the NHS 'waiting list dog' ever catch its tail? How in heaven's name can the needs of the increasing number of patients waiting to see a specialist ever be met?

The bigger mystery is that NHS managers are oblivious to this crucial phenomenon. The waiting list, when allowed to build up, is going to exponentially increase the waiting times for patients. You can either increase the number of doctors or stop people from falling ill. We have pointed out in the previous chapters that the NHS, which is unable to stop people from falling ill, is making every effort to reduce the number of patients requiring a specialist opinion from being referred by their GPs. In effect, the ingenious *NHS England, through the 'clinical commissioning groups'* is 'bribing' GPs not to send patients to the specialists! (We have provided details of this in the previous chapters.)

One cannot imagine a more pathetic and unsuccessful effort to reduce the waiting time for people in need of surgery or a specialist consultation.

The simple conclusion we have reached is that an exponentially growing waiting list causes problems that no amount of reactive cash injections can solve.

The only way to neutralise the awesome negative power of waiting lists, which can wreck any health care system, is by increasing the number of doctors.

We want to reiterate our firm belief that the doctors and nurses in the NHS are some of the best in the world; their knowledge, ability, dedication and expertise is second to none. Whenever we talk about the incompetence and inefficiency of the NHS, it relates to the management and NEVER the doctors or nurses.

The people living in the UK are lucky and blessed. Most of us have roofs over our heads, clean water, food and comfortable clothes that are available on demand.

Unfortunately, what is *not* available on demand and reasonably promptly is the ability to see a doctor if we develop a medical problem. In the UK, you should only fall ill during weekdays and strictly between 8am and 6pm, and, no, you cannot get an appointment with your GP unless you wait for 13 days (2.5 working weeks), if you are lucky. We have dealt with this issue in detail in previous chapters.

No new NHS model can work, as we are recommending it, unless some drastic changes are made to bring our Primary Care System close to what most other countries have to offer. This extraordinarily rotten system has a domino effect on the rest of the health service, as discussed previously.

Unable to get a GP appointment, people flock to A&E. In 2017, 64,782 people in England attended A&E every day. This means that people's attendance over one year was 23,645,430 (23.64 million) out of a total population of 55.26 million.

Out of 23,645,430 people seen in A&E, hospital admissions were 16,288 (yes, sixteen thousand two hundred and eighty-eight). This means that 23,629,142 people did not require hospital treatment. It is anyone's guess how many people out of the 23,645,430 had genuine accidents or were emergency cases.

We interviewed several A&E consultants extensively to find out what percentage of those attending could have been dealt with by their GPs. According to them, a large majority did not have to come in to see them and could have been treated by their GPs.

In late 2017 and early 2018, A&E admissions gathered momentum. As a result, 55,000 surgical procedures were cancelled, leaving hundreds of surgeons and nurses twiddling their thumbs in frustration. In 2016/17, overnight general and acute bed occupancy averaged 90.3% and regularly exceeded 95%. The internationally accepted safe occupancy bed level is 85%.

The two main problems requiring a solution are unacceptable delays to get GP appointments and non-availability of GP services after 6pm and over the weekends. The NHS's announcement to recruit 5000 more GPs, in our opinion, would only restore the numbers to pre-2012 levels. The number of GPs since Sept 2015 was down by 4.8%, to 27,773 in March 2018.

Our research shows an interesting phenomenon. The small number of single-handed GPs outperform most group practices in offering appointments to their patients, despite having a similar list to larger practices. The majority of the patients are able to get appointments in the same week and people can also walk in and be seen. It appears that the group practices have senior partners who conduct a minimum number of surgeries and let their junior-salaried or junior partners do most of the work. These partners seem to have several external interests, including membership of a CCG. Most group practices have female GPs, many of whom are mothers and have therefore chosen to work part-time.

We have a solution to this complex problem, without which the NHS would continue to be in a mess. We would increase the number of GPs and create a system of remuneration based on the number of patients seen in a week.

The GP's self-employed status would be abolished and changed to a salaried structure like their hospital colleagues, and all new GP vacancies and recruitment would be decided by the *Local NHS Centres*, of **NHS for us.**

The right of recruiting, exploiting and 'slave labouring' junior doctors at low wages by the longer-serving 'senior partners', and making vulgar amounts of money in the process, would also be abolished. Please remember that in 2015-16, 16 GPs in England made £300,000 to £800,000 and 193 made £200,000 to £300,000

In the new structure of 'NHS for us' every GP would be paid a basic wage, topped up by the number of patients seen each week. The current structure of a fixed yearly payment per patient would cease. A Minimum Acceptable Performance would be agreed for full and part-time GPs – the minimum number of patients that must be seen by the doctor per week. The financial rewards of every GP would be based on the number of patients seen.

Existing GP practices may retain the number of patients on their list for the sake of getting appointments, but patients would have the freedom to seek appointments with other GPs in the area, should their own practice doctors be unable to offer them one. A patient's medical records would be made available electronically to any other practice with the patient's consent. Our research shows that a majority of patients in a group practice do not see one specific GP all the time.

NHS managers have tried to come forward with the idea of giving choice to patients and creating an 'internal market', but this has had zero success and led to challenging consequences. Through our method, we have created a choice for the patients, who can contact any practice in the area to get an appointment if their own can't offer them one. In fact, there would be no guaranteed income for a GP for the privilege of having a patient on the list.

The new structure would provide incentives for GPs to see more patients, thus make more money. It would also give the patients new powers to become 'consultation seeking, money generating customers,' rather than being perceived as a nuisance.

The Bournemouth conference GPs would never want to 'turn away the patients', even if they were too busy, unless they wished to languish on a basic salary.

Over the next two years, online appointments with GPs would replace telephone consultations. Arrangements would be made for any GP to access the medical records of a patient from another practice electronically.

The planned NHS initiative to recruit an additional 5000 GPs is a good idea, but the number is not enough, as we will discuss in the following chapters. The *Local NHS Centre* of each region would undertake the recruitment process. We would recommend this recruitment from English-speaking countries, on a strict, non-renewable five-year visa.

PLAB examinations (these are tests to assess the suitability of a foreign graduate to practice in England) would distinguish between doctors wanting to be in general practice or a hospital specialist. Both parts of the exam would be held in doctors' own countries and visas would be provided to the suitable candidates. Those passing the exam and considered suitable for general practice would receive training from existing GPs.

Places for students to read medicine at UK universities would be increased threefold, and courses would be modified for doctors to specialise in general practice from day one. All doctors taught and funded by taxpayers would have to serve the NHS for a minimum period of seven years after graduation, excluding the period of training, in order to be allowed to practice as a GP. The **NHS for us** model would aim to generate a small but visible over supply of GPs in both the short and long-term.

We would change the current primary care coverage from 8am to 6pm to 11am to 8pm, with a final consultation at 7pm. This would have no cost implication. With fresh and new GPs, we would commence on a plan to offer GP services after hours and over the weekends.

The pathetic and 'ambulance dispatching' 111 services would be abolished. We have been unable to get the correct information, but, apparently, the contract cost is between £750 million to £1 billion.

Our recommendations would create a primary care system fit for the people of the UK, who would have the luxury of falling ill after 6pm and over the weekends. Most importantly,

A&E would be restored to a true Accident & Emergency Unit and not 'an out-of-hours GP service'. We have detailed plans on achieving this important aim, which is wrecking the entire hospital structure.

According to figures from NHS England, around 5000 people attend major A&E units more than 20 times each year. In 2016, they accounted for 3% of spending, which is £53 million. They probably account for a similarly outsized share of ambulance calls. **NHS for us** would severely curtail this abuse.

The worst NHS failing is in the suffering inflicted on people by making them wait to be seen by a hospital specialist or have a surgical procedure carried out. This has been the somewhat repetitive theme of this book (the waiting time to see a specialist was up from 18 weeks in 2017 to 22 weeks in 2018).

There has been a dangerous decline in the number of hospital beds available, which has been caused by the deliberate vandalism of NHS reformers in the name of saving money. Bed numbers have been steadily falling for over three decades. In 1987/88, NHS bed stock totalled 299,364 and fell to 142,568 in 2016/17, with the largest drop occurring in overnight mental health and learning disability facilities. These fell by 72.1% and 96.4%, respectively.

Official figures show that there was a drop of 12,000 beds between 2010 and 2016. Add to this a shortage of surgeons, specialists in all fields, especially psychiatrists, clinical psychologists, nurses and vital equipment, and the misery of the people requires no imagination to envisage.

The NHS has 2.7 beds per 1000 people, France 6.2/1000 and Germany 8.2/1000.

The most disturbing factor is the contradictory thinking of the NHS policy makers. Comrade (Sir) David Nicholson (CEO of the NHS, 2008-14) wanted centralisation and the closure of more hospitals. Jeremy Hunt, the outgoing health secretary, recently made a speech in which he said he wanted 10,000 more beds made available in the next few years.

It takes more than 15 years of postgraduate training for a doctor to become a consultant. NHS specialists in every field are as 'good as gold'. Our research indicates that over 50% of all surgeons have some input in private hospitals and 20-25% in other specialities.

We have already explained in detail that hospital consultants will have to make a choice between continuing to work in the NHS or resigning and going to work for the private hospital sector. The process of asking consultants to make a choice is likely to lead to opposition and unrest. Unfortunately, this has to be done. We simply cannot allow full-time consultants to work in competing private hospitals. We have detailed workable plans on how this can be achieved without causing an open rebellion.

The fact is that apart from a very small number of consultants working in London's NHS hospitals, no one is going to leave the prestigious, academically superb NHS to the 'isolation wilderness' of substandard private medical hotels. Above all, the annual income gleaned from private work at most non-London hospitals is never going to match the one from the NHS. One consultant physician we interviewed remarked, 'Private hospital income is the icing on the cake, but without the NHS cake, private hospital income is just the icing without the cake.'

Our research indicates a subconscious resentment and somewhat lowering of morale by those hospital consultants who have chosen not to work for private hospitals and who do not feel happy about working with 'burnt out' colleagues working extra to make money.

We interviewed several NHS consultants about why they had chosen not to work for a private hospital. A vast majority considered it a 'serious conflict of interest' and chose not to do so as a matter of conscience. Many consultants thought that working for private hospitals was a betrayal of the concept of the NHS by allowing the people with money to bypass the waiting lists.

One NHS consultant said, 'I could not sleep in peace at night while knowing that by receiving £200, I was seeing a patient whose counterpart, in a similar position, would be waiting five months to see me on the NHS.'

The greatest problem, which we have repeatedly brought to your attention, is the physical and mental anguish of people as their symptoms deteriorate whilst waiting months for an appointment.

We have explained, in detail, the consequence of an exponentially growing number of people waiting if only a small number of patients cannot be seen in a week. Our recommended plan is to have more than enough specialists and surgeons and to aim for *zero waiting*. Here is a brief summary of actions:

1. Recruit more specialists:
In January 2018, the number of hospital doctors in NHS England is 109,541. We feel that in order to achieve *zero waiting time*, we should budget to double the number of hospital doctors. Recruitment in the short to medium-term would be from the English-speaking countries, and the doctors selected would have already been working as top doctors in their speciality for more than five years and who possessed postgraduate qualifications. We advocate a five-year fixed work visa.

2. Increase the number of consultations and

surgical procedures:
This would be a process of synergistic agreement with hospital consultants in all specialities to see how each specialist could see more patients and perform more surgical operations every week. Our research indicates the willingness of a majority of hospital consultants to do more work, over the weekend and after hours, if they were provided with financial incentives to do so. This option was much favoured by the hospital doctors who were not working in private hospitals as a matter of choice and conscience.

3. Promote and upgrade senior registrars and registrars with postgraduate qualifications:
The NHS has a large pool of talented and experienced doctors who wait for a long time to be appointed as consultants. We advocate their urgent upgrades as consultants. In the short-term, senior consultants may supervise them.

4. Increase significantly the number of students in British universities:
This is the most neglected area by NHS planners. We believe the intake should be increased three times overall. Without this crucial action, the future of the NHS would depend on foreign doctors. Our research indicates that a very large number of students with excellent grades are currently being rejected due to a shortage of university places.

Up to now, we have talked almost exclusively

about GPs and hospital doctors. This is because we wanted to leave mention of hospital nurses to the end, like the best act in a variety show. We consider hospital nurses to be heroes, and unsung ones at that. It is the nurses who work in the most demanding and stressful conditions, and with such closeness to patients at all times. They work their hearts out and are treated with disrespect by unqualified managers who make them feel inadequate and unimportant. NHS managers have never got into their silly heads the crucial importance of nurses, who have seen their pay packets shrink. Our researchers were shocked to find one nurse regularly using a food bank to feed her family.

Nurses are viewed the same as any other member of staff in the army of 1.7 million people that the NHS employs. Their pay structure and pay rises are just like any other NHS worker.

We can provide you with page after page of statistics in every region in the UK, which reveal a massive shortage of nurses and one application for every 10 vacancies, including the constituency of our PM.

We have detailed plans for reversing this situation by first treating nurses as a different category of employee and giving them significant pay rises, boosting their status to similar to doctors.

In the short-term, we would give priority to

recruiting from abroad as many nurses as the NHS requires. In the medium term, we would run PR campaigns to attract the maximum number of applicants for nurse training via subsidised courses. We would ask for sponsorship from independent nursing home providers and employ specialists to alter nursing courses to make them shorter, if possible, and less academic and more practical. We would introduce a shorter course for care assistants and change their name to Associate Nurses at a higher salary than is currently being paid.

NHS for us, based in local hospitals, operating as *Local NHS Centres,* of the local People, by the local People, for the local People, is the future.

Chapter Fifteen

A Paradigm Shift
The first lesson of economics is scarcity;
there is never enough of anything free of any
value to fully satisfy all those who want it.
The first lesson of politics is to disregard
the first lesson of economics.

Please accept our apologies in advance for
repeating several points already made in previous
chapters. Here's what the researchers say about
remembering the written word;
"The 'Forgetting Curve' is steepest during the first
24 hours. Exactly how much you forget varies,
but much of it slips down the drain after the first
day, with more to follow in the days after, leaving
you with a fraction of what you took in. It is
like filling up a bathtub, soaking it in and then
watching the water run down the drain. It might
leave a film, but the rest is gone."

To quickly recap, we have established that the
inefficient and ineffective NHS business model is
the cause of every problem. The UK is the only
Western country where this 'centrally planned
economy', also called 'command economy', is
being practised, employing the largest number
of civilians by any government in the world: 1.7
million.

We have shown you that the NHS has created
a two-tier health service: A no waiting, instant-

treatment private hospital service for the rich and the misery of months of suffering for those who are not so rich. You have learned that the creation by the NHS of the private hospital sector, at the expense of taxpayers, is one of the biggest scandals of the century. The NHS provides rich NHS customers with free 24/7 support and treats complications that private hospitals with limited facilities are unable to. Worst of all, the NHS provides private hospitals with their fully employed consultants to treat rich patients by 'busting' the NHS queue. Private hospitals do not employ a single consultant, as there are none except those working in the NHS.

In previous chapters, we explained that in 2017/18, a staggering £147.5 billion, approximately 20% of total tax receipts, was allocated to the NHS. We have brought to your attention the breathtakingly incompetent and negligent practices of NHS managers and how vast sums of money are practically thrown in the bin. We have demonstrated that governments in power have never tried to find out what the real funding requirement of the NHS would be to achieve what every other European country has been achieving for years: a zero-waiting list and a zero annual financial deficit. Without doing this, the chance of the NHS being able to provide a first-class service is zero.

We have recommended decentralisation and the creation of *Local NHS Centres* based in each main regional hospital, with the allocation of all funds directly to them. We have given details on the structure of *Local NHS Centres* and how they would operate independently on a local level. (Chapter 12)

Spending hundreds of millions of pounds with the sole aim of distributing money to hospitals, pretending to buy services that the hospitals have been providing for years, makes no sense.

We advocated abolishing the 'clinical commissioning groups' their creator, NHS England, and the associated quangos. We are given to understand that the elimination of the so-called 'internal markets' and the cost involved in administering the monster would release anything from 20% to 30% of the entire NHS budget.

The most important point we brought to your attention was a very significant shortage of GPs, hospital doctors, nurses and equipment. Without wanting to be accused of being a conspiracy theorist, it is the shortage of doctors, nurses and equipment that produces horrendous waiting lists that then feed private hospitals with rich patients. We argued that in spite of NHS efforts to support private hospitals through means that are unfair and unjust, this sector would collapse if there were no waiting lists. Apart from billionaires and footballers, why would anyone spend money when free NHS treatment is available?

Our conclusive comment was that the government should come clean and tell taxpayers about the exact amount required for having enough doctors, nurses and equipment to create a zero-waiting list and a zero deficit. We feel that without the decentralisation and the abolition of the unsustainable and wasteful NHS infrastructure, the NHS could require £250 billion a year or more.

We are confident that implementing our proposals to decentralise and allow *Local NHS Centres* to fulfil the needs of the local community as **NHS for us,** is the only way to solve these NHS problems.

Unlike NHS reformists, we have a workable plan. We would develop and create a 'prototype' of Local NHS Centre in one hospital, which would be fully staffed with doctors, nurses and essential equipment to achieve zero-waiting lists.

New contracts would be made with GP's, specialists, surgeons on meeting a Minimum Performance Level of seeing a desired number of patients in a week and being paid a bonus per patient when this number is exceeded. (We have detailed proposals for this.). On successful completion this prototype, model would be copied and transferred to other *Local NHS Centres*

To summarise, we have brought to your attention WHAT is not working in the NHS, WHY the NHS is not working and HOW it can be changed to '**Put Patients First**'.

Until now, we haven't dared to bring to your attention a very important point, without which our recommended model probably won't work.

This requires a paradigm shift on your part and you need to read this story.

A dozen or so men and women were waiting for a train, which was late by more than an hour, on the platform of a small station with no waiting room. Five children, aged three to 10, were running a riot, much to the distress of the people waiting. The father of the children was sitting on his overcoat, on the floor, holding his head in his hands and oblivious to what his kids were doing. Ultimately, an elderly lady went up to the man and said, 'Can't you see how your kids are misbehaving? Are you not able to take control? Your kids are disturbing everyone here.' The rest of the crowd was pleased with this intervention.

The man suddenly stood up, his eyes red as if he had been crying, and said, 'Oh, I apologise. I am so sorry. You see, I have just come back from hospital where we went to see my terminally ill wife. She died while we were there.'

There was a stunned silence and within minutes everyone was attending to the children, giving them sweets and doing whatever they could do to help.

This is called a 'paradigm shift'.

Our final recommendations for the NHS require a paradigm shift of your own, which relates to the synonyms 'Free NHS' and 'Free for all NHS'.

What is totally free in the world and available to anyone? One example could be the internet. Companies make a fortune because a large number of people are able to access it. The other examples of 'free' things are, as you would expect, the air we breathe, natural beauty, the feel of sunshine or snow on our skin, quiet contemplation, conversation and a walk on the beach.

We looked for what is 'free for all'.

Collins Dictionary: British *'Free-for-all'*:
A disorganised brawl or argument, usually involving all those present.

Collins Dictionary: American *'Free-for-all'*:
A disorganised fight in which many take part; brawl.

Merriam Webster: Definition of *'Free-for-all'*:
A competition, dispute or fight open to all comers and usually with no rules.

Merriam Webster: Synonyms for *'Free-for-all'*:
Chaos, confusion, disarrangement, disarray, disorder, disorganisation.

In the UK, since 1948, *'Free-for-all'*: The NHS.

A 'free-for-all' NHS faithfully captures the meaning of the phrase, 'chaos, confusion, usually no rules, disorder, disorganisation'.

Here comes the paradigm shift: every person in the UK must pay a small amount to access any of the NHS services. This is not privatisation, as we will explain.

A 'free-for-all' NHS is unlikely to work, even with our recommendations. We are living in the fifth largest capitalist economy in the world, where every transaction is based on the exchange of money to buy or sell a service or product. We are all part of a society that creates wealth, either directly or indirectly. A person working in McDonald's on minimum wage is no less of a wealth creator than the chairman of a public company.

It is from the creation of this wealth that arises all the revenues for the state to spend on health, education and social benefit to those less privileged and in need. Every one of us (even those unemployed and on benefits) contributes to the economy by buying (or selling). There is nothing of financial value that is FREE in the world, except the NHS.

In our estimate, the NHS provides no service that has a value of less than one hundred pounds sterling. And it is free; you can see your GP as often as you want, go to A&E as many times as you wish, be referred to see a specialist whenever required or ring 999 and have an ambulance come and get you as often as you need. Free-for-all.

The NHS was one of the first of its kind in providing universal health care to its people. The concept was refined and is now successfully in existence in most European countries, with one main difference. The health care in these countries is not *free-for-all*. A health insurance system exists, where each individual has to take responsibility for their health by paying a small amount, with no one allowed to opt out.

We hasten to add that the European health insurance system bears no resemblance to the notorious US health insurance system, where over 10% of Americans are uninsured and a majority of personal bankruptcy cases are due to inability to pay medical bills. The US does not have a universal health care system. For over a decade, the CEO of *NHS England* Simon Stevens was the boss of UnitedHealth, one of the largest health insurance companies in the US.

The UK public is right to be wary of the health insurance system practised in the US. Let it not be compared with the same system in most European countries. First, the health care covers everyone; second, the premium is very small, 'a tiny fraction of the cost'; third, the premium would never go up, no matter how much a person's ill health may demand. Lastly, everyone can afford it.

The principal established by European countries is not that governments need public money to provide a universal health care system, but rather that by contributing a small amount of money every person is made responsible for looking after his/her own health and contributing to the health fund.

We have conducted extensive research and developed a fundamental structure of financial participation by the public. It is not a health insurance scheme. The main features of our 'direct financial input' by the UK people are as follows:

1 Everyone living in the UK must pay, without exception, a small sum to access any of the medical services at all times.

2 The payment amount by the British public would be in keeping with what people are paying in other EU countries. In reality, it would be considerably less.

3 The principal of universal health care would be strictly maintained, with a cap on the maximum amount that would ever be spent by an individual in one calendar year.

In order to determine the equitable yearly health budget that every person in the UK must allow for, let us look at some aspects of health provision across the world. A report published in December 2017 by the World Bank and the World Health Organisation found that half of the world's population does not have access to essential health services. More than 800 million people spend over 10% of their annual household income on medical expenses; nearly 180 million spend over 25%.

We decided to examine the spending patterns of the 'British household', as provided by the Office for National Statistics, for the year ending 2017:

Recreation & culture	£73.50/week
Restaurants & hotels	£50.10/ week
Clothing & footwear	£25.10/week
Alcohol drinks	£11.90/week

Before you, the reader, decide if our proposed charges are fair, please don't forget that money spent on 'recreation, culture, restaurants and hotels' by a British household is £123.60 per week.

Contrary to the belief held by most people, not every service provided by the NHS is free, and an increasing number are paid for. In 1951, only three years after the creation of the NHS, a charge was made for use of NHS dentistry services. The most interesting aspect of these charges is that except for those under 18, almost everyone has to pay – the over 60s and those on employment benefits, etc. In most personal circumstances, where the NHS provides an exemption from a charge, the NHS dentistry service does not.

We would like to bring to your attention a list of

NHS dentistry charges as of 1st April 2018:

Operation	Charge
Band one	£21.60
Band two	£59.10
Band three	£256.50
Fitting of dentures	£256.00

The prescription charge for each item that your GP prescribes is £8.80 from April 18, 2018.

Eye tests costs £21.31, single vision lenses cost £70.00 and each contact lens is £57.

We recommend a weekly budget of £8/week for every person over a 12 months period, with a capping mechanism so that someone *never pays more than a certain amount* in any calendar year.

We recommend the following three payment bands, which is the same system NHS dentistry has been using since 1951, only considerably cheaper(see table on the following page):

Band	Amount	Facilities
A	£10	GP visit Blood tests X-ray Ambulance call Minor injury walk-in clinics Daily hospital bed charge for four days in-patient treatment. Please note that Band A of NHS dentistry costs £21.60. You may be interested to know that a vet charges £35-40 per consultation for a dog or cat.
B	£20	A&E attendance Hospital Specialist consultation MRI or CT scan Daily hospital bed charge on the fifth day of hospitalisation. Please note that Band B of NHS dentistry costs £59.10. The average emergency charge by a vet for a dog or cat is £150-£1500.
C	£50	Surgical procedure. NHS dentistry in Band C costs £256.50. The average surgical procedure of a dog or a cat under general anaesthetics is £3000-£4500.

Let us examine the projected cost of a year's access to medical services by one person, with just £8/week at a budget of £416 a year.

In one calendar year, if a person has eight GP consultations, calls an ambulance twice, visits A&E once, sees a specialist once, has one blood test and one MRI scan, the total amount comes to £170.

An additional surgical operation under general anaesthetic would be £50. Add to it a four-day stay in hospital and it comes to £90; the grand total is, therefore, £260 for this almost maximum use of NHS services by an average person.

Giving a conservative estimate, the cost to the NHS for providing this set of services would be £5,000 to £10,000.

Our proposed charges would be applicable to everyone, with no exception.

People in full-time employment and those self-employed and paying a basic rate of tax would be capped at a maximum of £8/week. This means that if and when the £416 limit was reached, there would be no further charge.

In keeping with the system of NHS dentistry charges, people over 60 and those unemployed and on benefits would still have to pay, but their fees could be capped at £4/week at £208 in one calendar year. Under 18s may be capped at £1 /

week at £52 in a calendar year.

The fundamental principal here is a paradigm shift, where budgeting a small amount of money for NHS services becomes a symbol of taking responsibility for one's own health. We strongly advocate that there cannot be any exemptions. Everyone must pay for accessing any NHS service.

The principal of the British public making a small contribution to access health services would help prevent the NHS being used as the free ATM machine. Currently, anyone can draw out any amount at any time, without ever having contributed to the UK taxation system.

Our pathetic and feeble politicians have turned the NHS into 'charity for all' in order to gain the UK a reputation as a compassionate and caring country.

A recent order by the government warned all GPs to register everyone and provide suitable treatment, without them being required to identify as British taxpayers. Our well-informed researchers suggest that health tourism costs the NHS, on average, £1.8 billion a year.

During our research and interviews, we were appalled to hear stories of people on visitor visas giving the address of a relative or renting an English apartment and obtaining free antenatal care and delivering their babies in NHS hospitals, with the added benefit of the child being born as a

British national.

At a time when the NHS is collapsing from a shortage of funds, rich people from other countries fly to the UK for free treatment. The leaders of the NHS appear to take pride and delight in these idiotic philanthropic policies. Our proposed *Local NHS Centres* of **NHS for us** would never allow these.

According to the OBR (Office for Budget Responsibility), the 'accelerating cost of the NHS will double the national debt, relative to the GDP, by mid century.'

We are confident that the proposed model of '**NHS for us**' is the only way to provide a credible health service that the UK economy can afford. Several politicians and analysts want to raise money by increasing tax. The problem with this kind of taxation is that the extra revenue generated does not always go to the NHS but gets gobbled up by the treasury for other matters. A 'free-for-all' system creates unlimited demands and stops people from taking responsibility for their own health.

A recent poll by the independent think tank Reform indicates a shift of opinion amongst the British public. The need to have prompt and easy access to NHS services is so paramount that: 'to 64% of the voters, it does not matter whether hospitals or surgeries are run by the government, not-for-profit organisations or the private sector.'

The proposed model of '**NHS for us**', which would make people pay a fraction of what the NHS costs, is a radical and welcome departure to bring the UK health service in line with other European countries, where people have to make a significantly more financial contribution towards looking after their health.

Devolving the responsibility of health care management to local level and abolishing the 'internal markets' and all quangos, including *NHS England*, and allowing people to contribute a very small sum towards using NHS services would solve most problems and produce the crucial zero-waiting lists and zero financial deficit.

NHS for us, based in local hospitals, operating as *Local NHS Centres,* of the local People, by the local People, for the local People.

Chapter Sixteen

Let us wake to a new dawn

BBC and Sky journalists jointly commented:
'The big story is not that the NHS needs more money to stay afloat, the real issue is that no one is prepared to recognise that it needs to be run differently if it is to survive.'

The ultimate conclusion of this book is to change the NHS in its present format and run it differently, through a new model – '**NHS for us**' – with one guiding principle, one goal:
To have zero waiting lists and zero financial deficit at all times – and to 'Put Patients First.'

In the 70 years of its existence, the NHS has failed every year to achieve the above objective. The horrendous waiting time for patients and the resulting physical and mental anguish have been the main subject of this book and it's been repeated often.

We are providing answers to these dual problems.

Zero waiting periods to access any NHS service:
One of the most important findings of our 18-months of research is this:
Most GPs, every hospital specialist and every surgeon treat fewer patients in a week than is required, leading to exponentially growing numbers of patients every week, building a longer and longer queue, for which the NHS has no

solution.

The only answer is to have more doctors and to explore how they can be incentivised to see more patients. This can be achieved by the mutual agreement of a 'Minimum Performance Level'. Financial incentives would be put in place after the Minimum Performance has been met. We have detailed plans for it.

The number of GPs in March 2018 totalled 27,773. We feel that the NHS requires minimum of **15,000 more** GP's to be able to ensure no waiting and an additional service to provide after hours and weekend cover.

The number of hospital doctors in January 2018 totalled 109,541. We advocate a minimum number of **100,000 more** specialists and surgeons.

The number of nurses in January 2018 totalled 286,215. The NHS needs a minimum of **120,000 more** nurses.

The need to replace and update diagnostic and other equipment is urgent, as it will save the NHS money and avoid it sending patients to private 'for profit' hospitals, all of which make a killing. Freedom of information research indicates that equipment critical to early diagnosis and the treatment of cancer is decades old. Here are some figures:

892 X-ray machines are more than 10 years old;

139 are past their replacement dates.

295 ultrasound machines are more than 10 years old; 134 are past their replacement dates.

46 MRI scanners are more than 10 years old; 10 are past their replacement dates.

45 CT scanners are more than 10 years old; 10 are past their replacement dates.

The NHS has fewer CT scanners – 8 per million – compared to the EU average of 21.4 and fewer MRI scanners – 6.1 million – compared to the EU average of 15.4.

Zero Financial Deficit: Let us see what the cost would be of recruiting more doctors, nurses and purchasing equipment.

GPs: 15,000 more may cost £2 billion.

Hospital Doctors: 100,000 more may cost £10 billion.

Nurses: 120,000 more may require £6 billion.

Equipment: Initial budget, £2 billion.

To sum up the above, the NHS in England requires a projected additional £20 billion annually to produce a zero-waiting time for patients and zero financial deficit. More calculations would be required to find out the additional cost for Scotland, Wales and Northern Ireland.

Our conclusion is that the country is unable to provide an additional £20 billion annually for NHS England alone, especially when considering the NHS's historic financial mismanagement record. Our proposed solution is to turn the old, unworkable NHS into a new model. '**NHS for us**' which will achieve the dual goals, without bankrupting the country.

The shortfall would be achieved as follows:
Savings from dismantling NHS England and its quangos and abolishing the 'internal markets' purchasers/providers scam = £8 billion.

(Several analysts believe that eliminating the so-called 'internal markets' scenario alone could save 20% or more of the budget allocation.)

Revenue from contribution by people using '**NHS for us**' services = £8 billion.

Savings from wasteful NHS spending = £5 billion.

Total savings = £21 billion, and these could be even more.

We are confident that the new model, '**NHS for us**', will save enough money to not require more from the government, while creating zero waiting times and zero deficit at all times.

A summary of our proposed list of actions is as follows:

1. Decentralisation and devolution of the NHS clinical, financial and general management to 150 or more regional hospitals:
Major hospitals have been providing inpatient, outpatient, diagnostic and A&E services to a geographically based local community of 275,000 to 500,000 people each for decades, and they cover the entire of England. These centres of excellence employ some of the best specialists, surgeons and nurses in the world. Our new model **NHS for us,** proposes that each of the major regional hospitals would be made independent from the clutches of remote central managers, to look after the needs of the local community. These would be named *Local NHS Centres*. Please refer to Chapter 12 for details.

2. The dismantling of NHS England, and all its related quangos: The communist-inspired, 'central command economy' management structure of the NHS, which employs the largest number of people by a government in the world and is run in England by the wasteful, autocratic, unaccountable, inefficient, ineffective *NHS England*, would be dismantled. The NHS funds would go directly to all *Local NHS Centres*.

3. The NHS 'internal markets' would be abolished: The concept of 'purchaser' and 'provider' within the NHS monopoly would cease. Nobel Prize-winning economists Maskin, Myerson and Hurwicz, said, 'You cannot rely on market forces to provide quality health care.

Sellers have an incentive to seek the highest possible sale price and buyers have the opposite incentive.'

4. Everyone using any NHS service would make a small payment; no exemptions: The amount paid would be small and affordable, with a cap on the maximum amount a person would ever spend over a 12-month calendar period.

The financial contribution made by a person would *never increase* because of more use of medical services.

*5. Every company in the UK, on line or otherwise, offering medical advice, service or treatment would be **regulated**.* Details in chapter 17.

All measures would be taken to safeguard and enhance the financial rewards and job satisfaction of GPs, hospital doctors and nurses, to make them the true heroes of '**NHS for us**'. The abolition of 'internal markets' would make it possible to eliminate toxic bureaucratic paperwork, which vastly reduces the contact time between doctors/nurses and patients.

Research conducted by the NHS Confederation shows that clinical staff spend up to 10 hours a week collecting or checking data, and that more than one third of the work is neither useful nor relevant to patient care. It is estimated that collecting this data alone costs the NHS £500 million. This useless practice would be reviewed and abolished.

The details of decentralisation of the NHS and devolution to regional hospitals acting as independent Local NHS Centres has been provided in chapter 12.

Though the charitable Local NHS Centres would operate independently, they would work together and have a non-bureaucratic and charitable, body, which could be named 'Coordination Centre'

This would be a benign, self-regulatory organisation, which would coordinate the activities of each centre and ensure maintenance and enhancement of clinical standards and any problems a Local NHS Centre is facing. The 'Coordination Centre' would join forces with charitable think tank giants like The King's Fund, the Health Foundation, the Institute for Fiscal Studies, the Nuffield Trust to have their researchers' insights in to improving all aspects of the Local NHS Centres.

Procedures would be developed for 'continuous improvement', through feedback of patients, doctors, nurses and other staff.

Great emphases would be put in participation of the local people and communities, to form supportive volunteer groups specially to rectify the concerns of patients and their relatives.

The big advantage of every Local NHS Centre as

a charitable organisation is that it would attract and work with other charities to convey messages about keeping good health and trying to prevent lifestyle-induced disease. Local radio, TV and print media would work together to produce a feeling of pride and achievement in the workings of the Local NHS Centre. There would be little need to spend millions to convey a message to own community.

We have extensive plans, to make **NHS for us** a truly great organisation, from a faceless NHS run by remote managers to a warm, personal organisation, with zero waiting time to access any medical service and a zero financial deficit.

Let us wake to a new dawn and throw away the shackles of 70 years of an NHS run by incompetent managers.

Welcome to **NHS for us,** of the local People, by the local People, for the local People.

Chapter Seventeen

What can be cured must NOT be endured

Publication of the book was delayed to allow the addition of this chapter.

As this book was sent for publication, there came the news that Matt Hancock the new Health Secretary had announced, in his public speech, that he had joined Babylon, stating:
"My GP is through the NHS on Babylon Health, it's brilliant".

This has led to so much controversy, especially in the medical press, that our advisers asked us to investigate the growing role of Private General Practice in the UK, in particular the consequences of the health secretary joining Babylon and include our findings in this book.

We have delayed the publication of the book to do so and this special chapter has been added.

You may remember that in chapter two, we exposed the Private Hospital Sector to be a 'scam' and proved that in reality it is a wholly created, supported and dependent parasite of the NHS.

It is becoming clear that the NHS General Practice is now sliding towards the 'scam' similar to the Private Hospital sector. Profit making companies are offering Private GP appointments.

The existence of a two-tier health care system

in the UK that we discussed in chapter one, in relation to the Private Hospital Sector, is now being rapidly expanded to General Practice. The rich can see a GP privately within 24 hours whilst NHS patients must wait for 2 weeks or more.

Several 'for-profit' companies have mushroomed. Their Mission Statement is:
"We bust the NHS GP waiting period by offering immediate private appointments to the wealthy and make huge profits for our shareholders"

Private Health Insurance companies lining up to offer this service are; HCA Healthcare UK, BUPA, Nuffield Health, Vitality Health.

Not to be left behind, private hospitals like Spire Health Care, BMI Health Care, Nuffield Hospitals, Ramsay Health Care have joined the field. Virgin Healthcare has thrown its hat into the ring too.

Lesser known companies like Doctalay, GPDQ, Push Doctor, Babylon, Summerfield Healthcare have also joined the fray.

We decided to explore in detail the workings of Babylon, of which the health secretary Matt Hancock, is a patient.

Babylon Healthcare Services Ltd, was incorporated on 22 Sept.2014, company no. 09229684, with two directors, Dr. Ali Parsadoust and Mr. C.W. Bischoff.

Publicly available company accounts showed the net worth of the company in the year ending 2015 was £11,409 (Eleven thousand four hundred nine). This jumped up to £126,286, *according to accounts, for the year ending 2016.* Accounts for 2017 and for 2018 are still to be submitted, at the time of this book going to publication.

We found it interesting to note that a company worth less than £12,000 in 2015 and less than £127,000 in 2016 should claim on its website by its founder and CEO Ali Parsa that: "Babylon is home to the largest collection of scientists, clinicians, mathematicians and engineers".

It may come as a surprise to hear that the aforementioned founder and CEO of Babylon Healthcare Services Ltd., Mr. Ali Parsa, was also the founder and CEO of Circle Holdings, the first private company to manage a NHS hospital (Hinchingbrooke) and which proved to be a spectacular failure.

At the time of taking over a 10 year contract to manage the hospital, Mr. Ali Parsa, criticising the management of the NHS commented: "If Healthcare was an airline, we are losing a 747 every year. We have nothing like quality control, we have nothing like the productivity and efficiency gains that other industries have".

His company, Circle Holdings, was supposed

to be the John Lewis partnership of Healthcare, with staff shareholding and involved in decision making. This never materialised. In 2012 the company was failing and staff morale was at its worst.

The newspaper headlines shouted, "Circle says it is driven by its patients – but it's been looking rather sick by itself." The Care Quality Commission inspected Hinchingbrooke hospital and found "patients being neglected, poor hygiene and staffing problems".

Mr. Ali Parsa, the founder and chief executive of Circle, seeing the writing on the wall and having spectacularly failed in his promises, resigned.

Tracy Lambert, the head of health for UNISON, said "Mr. Ali Parsa is walking away. He made a lot of claims about the unprecedented level of savings he could make. Not only are these claims exaggerated, but they are made at the expense of staff and patients".

Circle Holdings abandoned its 10 year contract to manage the Hinchingbrooke hospital after only two years, leaving the hospital in a big financial and management mess.

The latest Care Quality Commission Report was published it appears in the afternoon, after the morning announcement of withdrawal of Circle from the contract. The report stated Hinchingbrooke hospital to be 'Inadequate

<u>Overall'</u> and specifically for 'patient safety and leadership'.

Most damning, it was the first hospital trust that the watchdog had ever found to be 'Inadequate' in all areas and that had been placed in 'special measures'.

The only beneficiary of this disastrous exercise was Mr. Ali Parsa CEO and founder of Circle and now the CEO and founder of Babylon. According to The Guardian and this is reproduced exactly as it was reported:
"In 2012, his final year as chief executive, Parsa was paid £1.1m. As well as £415,000 salary he received £564,000 linked to the end of his contract, comprising £400,000 salary, a £71,000 termination payment and £85,000 towards his pension."

With the history of delusional and failed statements by the founder and CEO Mr. Ali Parsa, no one can take seriously his pronouncement on Babylon that "a chatbot can diagnose a medical condition as accurately as a GP". The medical profession has condemned this nonsense unanimously.

Babylon Healthcare states on its website:
"Babylon's mission is to put an accessible and affordable health services in the hands of every person on earth. With existing operations in the UK and **Rwanda**, we are on the path to achieving

our goals (plus plans in progress with major providers in China, USA and the Middle East)".

Whilst we have been unable to trace any operational activity of Babylon in China, the US or the Middle East, we considered it prudent to take a look at the only country the company considered fit to start its operations – Rwanda.

Rwanda, came to the attention of the world in 1994 when an estimated 500,000 to 1,000,000 people were killed, notoriously called Rwanda Genocide. The African country is not exactly a next-door neighbour of the UK. The minimum flight times for the only direct flights are 9 hours 40 minutes from Gatwick and 11 hours 15 minutes from Heathrow.

A major UK newspaper headline on 24thJuly 2017 lamented:
"Britain gives £64 million in foreign aid to despot Rwanda dictator."

Mr. Paul Kagame has been the president of the country since 2000 and through a change in constitution can stay as president till 2034. The African country is small in size, world's 149th out of 192 countries.

According to fdu-rwanda.com on 21st Feb. 2018, The Freedom House report in 2016 considers "Rwanda a 'non-free' country with a score of 8/40 in terms of political and human rights".

Our big question and a very valid one too, is this: Why did Babylon start its operations in Rwanda, a 10-11 hours flight away from the UK and ruled since the year 2000, by an oppressive dictator with a bad human rights record and a mandate to continue as president until 2034?

We have checked Babylon's activities in this small third world African country and they are not for charity.

Let us look then at the operations of Babylon. We will not concern ourselves at this stage with the company's private online consultations nor Mr. Ali Parsa's histrionics about its chatbot being as accurate in diagnosis as a doctor.

We have investigated the involvement of Babylon with the NHS. It appears that any NHS patient can join the General Practice of Babylon by first de-registering with their own GP. Babylon will then be paid £150 annually by the NHS for looking after the patient.

However, if you are suffering from certain medical problems, you cannot join Babylon. These conditions are: pregnancy, adults with safeguarding needs; people with complex mental health conditions; people with complex physical, psychological, social needs; those with dementia, older people with conditions related to frailty; people requiring end of life care; parents of children who are on the 'Child at Risk' register;

people with learning disabilities and people with drug dependence.

This shows without any shadow of a doubt that Babylon NHS services are only available to persons who are healthy and without chronic or challenging medical conditions. Those in need of regular medical attention cannot join Babylon.

The Pareto principal of 80:20 applies in General Practice; 80 percent of patients require 20% or less GP time whilst the other 20% require 80% or more GP time.

Imagine now that 80% of patients of a GP practice, a bit fed up with the waiting time to see their own GP a few times a year, decide to switch to Babylon or similar companies for 'instant appointments'. The NHS GP would suddenly find their income reduced by 80% whilst doing the same amount of work to provide medical services to those most in need. The GP practice would no longer be a viable proposition and would be forced to close.

The new Health Secretary Matt Hancock's decision to join a company like Babylon to provide his NHS GP services and then to announce his support of the company, has demonstrated his total ignorance of the basics of the NHS.

It is unacceptable to have a health secretary, who doesn't have a clue about the Universal Health

Care system that the NHS has been providing since 1948. By joining Babylon, he has accepted that the NHS General Practice can choose to provide healthcare to people comparatively free from symptoms and refuse to offer GP services to those in regular need and challenging physical or mental health conditions.

This shameful process of cherry picking represents a serious breach in the fundamental principles of the NHS.

The Health Secretary has publicly supported Babylon's intentions to lure NHS patients with minimum health needs and refuse those with chronic and challenging medical conditions. We believe that he is unfit to continue in this important post. His ignorance about the disastrous financial consequences of this process to NHS General Practices, makes his position untenable.

Upset by discovering the unethical practices of Babylon used to dupe the naïve health secretary Matt Hancock, we decided to find out where companies like Babylon were recruiting the new GPs from.

What category of doctors would provide the next day private GP appointments working for a private company? Were these junior hospital doctors with no general practice experience? Had these doctors been recruited from abroad, without

UK general practice expertise?

NHS GPs surely could not be providing this service, as we know the national average waiting list to secure a GP appointment is 2 weeks.

Worried that inexperienced doctors were working for the private companies, we wanted to investigate and find out.

What we discovered is shocking; all the private appointments are being provided by the existing NHS GPs!

Read my lips, there are no GPs hired by these companies from any other source; they all work as GPs in the NHS.

This must be nipped in the bud and stopped through our regulatory policy.

The new model of NHS described in detail in chapters 11-15, **NHS for us** would regulate every private company offering medical services to the public.

NHS for us would create a new department to offer compulsory registration to every company online or offline, every clinic, every hospital offering simple or complex medical services or advice to the British public.

One of our researchers moaned whilst studying organisations which offer medical services to the public in the UK, with no need to register or necessity to undergo any scrutiny into its ethics and expertise, "it's a jungle out there".

REGULATORY DETAILS

Companies offering online or offline medical services, medical advice, offer of prescriptions or similar would have to register and procure a 'Licence to operate'. A company like Babylon, which offers to provide GP services but refuses to accept NHS patients by discriminating against them on the grounds of existing medical conditions (no matter how complex and challenging), would not be granted a licence.

Private clinics and private hospitals would have to register. A group owning a number of hospitals or clinics would register each clinic or hospital individually.

Wealthy persons, queue busting in order to seek next day GP appointments and instant hospital specialists' consultations, would not be allowed to use any of the NHS diagnostic, treatment and other facilities for a period of three months from the date of commencement of private treatment. They would be required to use the facilities of the private clinics and hospitals.

The companies providing private medical services would need to supply a list of doctors offering their service with CVs, as a part of the registration process. No new doctor appointment would be made without submitting a CV for approval. A doctor considered unsuitable to provide services would not be employed.

A doctor employed by the NHS full time or part time, could not be employed by a private company, offering medical services to the public. All such doctors would need to be exclusively employed by the private company.

We need to explain in more detail the proposed regulatory process of the multibillion pound Private Hospital Industry.

Every hospital would be required to mirror the facilities of a standard regional NHS hospital and a Regulatory Inspection Team would scrutinise it. A referral to an NHS hospital to admit a patient that the private hospital was unable to deal with, would lead to an immediate suspension of the licence, followed by permanent cancellation if the private hospital was unable to prove its independence in dealing with all complications and botched operations.

We have already pointed out that any company offering private medical (or surgical) services could not employ doctors working part time or full time in the NHS and a list of all doctors would have to be made available to the Regulatory Authorities.

In the previous chapters, **NHS for us,** we explained that General Practice would be regulated. GPs' self-employed status would be abolished, and they would be salaried doctors like their hospital colleagues. The wheeling and dealing by greedy doctors to create super practices and make millions at the expense of the taxpayers, would cease. GPs providing same day services and seeing more patients would be financially rewarded and would be significantly better off than those with minimal contact with the patients and have converted NHS general practice into a money-making machine.

A challenge to anyone suggesting that the proposed regulation of private companies is unfair or unjust. (Please remember these apply only to services provide by the doctors).

The NHS allows unethical individuals and unregulated companies to operate without providing any evidence of the quality of services they provide, therefore putting vulnerable patients at risk. They can make unsubstantiated claims, verging on quackery, with no accountability.

If the Regulatory Mechanisms advocated were in place, people with a history of making delusional false statements, like Mr. Ali Parsa in the case of Circle Holdings, would have to undergo fairly stringent 'evidence-based tests' to prove the validity of the claims made by Babylon, before granting a licence.

We have learned of stories where cosmetic operations undertaken by ill trained surgeons in small private clinics have gone horribly wrong for patients. The five-star, ill equipped medical hotels posing as private hospitals have been making billions for years. We have no objection to them offering their services to the wealthy people. However, through the proposed regulations, they would no longer be allowed to steal services of super qualified specialists, surgeons or GPs fully employed by the NHS and offer them money to work part time.

No longer would the NHS provide free emergency admissions to the 'queue busting' rich patients when the private medical hotels are unable to cope, due to the pathetic absence of their own facilities.

No longer would the private GP companies be allowed to accept 'healthy' NHS patients and refuse those with existing physical or mental conditions, as supported by the new Health Secretary, Matt Hancock.

No longer would the wealthy patients be allowed to have NHS prescriptions, diagnostic tests or treatment free on NHS. They would need to wait for a period of three months from the time of commencing private treatment.

Are these proposed regulations, the results of a 'leftists loony, rich bashing policy'? Not at all. The NHS has created a two-tier healthcare system in the UK; private GPs and private hospitals offer instant treatment to the rich, leaving the rest to wait on the NHS.

These regulations would produce an even playing field. The rich can continue to smash the ordinary folks' NHS queues. The private hospitals and private GP companies can continue to make their billions but **NOT**, definitely **NOT** by using the NHS doctors nor free NHS facilities.

We challenge anyone to prove us wrong.

Epilogue

Go, set a watchman, let him declare what he seeth

Most writers want to share their thoughts, their stories and their philosophy. They have an inner urge to communicate – perhaps for the fame or maybe for the money. Great books produce a bang, the less fortunate ones a whimper. They all end up forgotten, some gathering dust in libraries, others waiting to be 'kindled'.

The author of this book, along with the doctors, nurses, advisers and researchers he's worked with, has no such lofty ambitions. This book is a message of hope and salvation to the millions suffering and the many millions more who do not know what will happen when they need medical attention. This book is a platform for starting a national campaign of awareness and change in order to 'Put Patients First'.

The NHS is a multibillion, money making machine for the ever increasing 'for profit companies', but this comes at the expense of the British taxpayer. Private health insurance enterprises, private medical hotels pretending to be hospitals, profit greedy companies from the US, and tax havens are the vultures. These dark forces, working in full co-operation with the biggest quango in the world, NHS England, are threatening the very existence of the NHS.

One of the ways to bring about change in the

NHS can be with the agreement of political parties to amend and produce new legislation. Initially, this could prove difficult because the deficiencies of the NHS provide strong evidence to the opposition of the failures of the government, which they can utilise as a platform to help them win the next election.

The solution to solve all the NHS's ills, put forward by the _government_ appears to involve allowing 'for profit companies' to cherry pick clinical and other services, without understanding that the purchaser/provider concept in healthcare does not work. As long ago as 2007, Nobel Prize winners Maskin, Myerson and Hurwicz concluded through the _Mechanism Design Theory_ that:
'Because sellers have an incentive to seek the highest possible sale price and buyers have the opposite incentive, both parties have different levels of knowledge about the overall value of the transaction. As a result, the final result may not be efficient. You cannot rely on market forces to provide quality health care.'

The Labour party believes a larger cash injection would help, and the Liberal Democrats think a pence increase in tax would make all the difference. The NHS is the beautiful game of political football and no party seems remotely interested in a radical reform process. Worse of all, none are aware of the waiting times people face.

All of us need to work together to bring about change in the NHS. In order to make this happen, the people of the UK need to get together and demand it. A massive amount of money is being spent on providing a third-world health service, in spite of the NHS having the best doctors and nurses in the world. To fight and succeed against these formidable opponents who could stand to lose a fortune is no easy task.

We need your help. It is a battle of people versus quangos; people versus multibillion corporations; people versus the government; the health of the nation versus vested interests. We are confident that with your help and participation, David will defeat Goliath.

When victory comes, you won't have to wait for weeks to see your GP, five to six months to consult a specialist, and seven to 12 months to have a surgical procedure. If the rest of Europe can do it, so can we.

Please join us to change what must be changed.

www.nhsisnotworking.com

dr.hs@nhsisnotworking.com

Amazon Reviews First Edition
from Verified Purchasers

We all know that there are failings within the NHS system-if this was a private business it would have been bankrupt many years ago.

Things have changed in the world of care and in business but the NHS hasn't moved far enough with the times.

This book is both insightful and thought provoking. It is written by a doctor who knows the issues behind the scenes. As a nurse myself I had views on the NHS (which we are obviously grateful for - but it does need bringing up to date).

A MUST READ for anyone interested in health, NHS and / or politics.

The Author as a health professional working in the care sector for some years has spent a great deal of time and effort gathering the information contained in this book. It is easy to read, with lots of facts and figures. I had mixed emotions as I read through each section . It opens your eyes to what happens daily and explains why waiting lists are so long. I have witnessed my own family members in severe pain waiting months for treatments, their quality of life taken from them as they deteriorated. The NHS clearly needs management comprised from Drs and nurses (the people that actually care) and not the government who neither care, understand or are interested in the well being of their own people. The proposals to move forward and save our NHS outlined in this book are fair and have been thought about with all considerations to every individual. I believe our younger generations will be the ones who suffer if changes are not made and I would recommend everyone, especially those with children to read this book.

I know that in the age of politicians such as Trump and Gove we are supposed to think that facts and experts don't mean much. But they do. They really do. Because facts, statistics and empirical evidence provide the solid foundation for making life and death decisions. And that is the case with this book by Dr. Sarwar, who has worked within the system for a long time and, therefore, knows its smallest nooks and crannies very intimately. Its prose may have been crafted a bit better but the greatest strength of the book, apart from its readability - such a fresh contrast to the turgid and dry approach of many of its ilk - is its Gatlin gun approach to facts. This book would give new ammunition (pun fully intended) even to seasoned campaigners. I, for instance, had no idea that private hospitals in the country do not employ any of their own doctors and that all doctors working in them are employed in the NHS. The extent of moonlighting and conflict of interest that the book highlights, are a shock to the system and meant to jolt us out out of our complacency that "our NHS is the best in the world." It is not. The best compliment I can pay is to say that this is the book I would read a day before going to a public consultation meeting on the NHS. With its wealth of fingertip evidence it is a must have for anyone interested in saving the NHS.

This is a well written expose of the inner workings of the NHS, explaining somewhat the never ending crises of the NHS. I was taken aback about the nature of the relationship between the private and NHS sectors. You can become overwhelmed by all the statistics thrown at you, but I suppose that is like the NHS behemoth itself.

An engrossing read, you will be better equipped to deal with the NHS if you find yourself regularly requiring the NHS.

Furthermore, next time there's a political furore about the dismantling of the NHS, you'll have some context and inconvenient truths that you know must be addressed eventually.

Just as this book has been published the current news includes yet further praise and government funding of for the NHS at the same time as one NHS Trust is reputedly 'privatising' elective orthopaedic surgery to a private company. This book is essential reading for any person who wants to see stark, accurate and well researched facts and figures to counteract the myths about the NHS that are so often repeated that they are treated as if they were facts.

Dr Sarwar lets the facts speak for themselves: the abuses of funding; the strange system of private consultants paid by the NHS; the inefficiencies of a centralised bureaucracy; the long waits to see doctors. All of this is backed up by examples and statistics.

This book starts the conversation for reform, but there is a mountain to climb in changing public opinion, where every political party treats the NHS as the organisation that dare not be criticised. The information is there to justify the criticisms. This book deserves a wide readership

Dr Sarwar gives a lot of detail of what goes wrong in the NHS and where and why; If tempted to give up reading the lists, skip to chapter sixteen, which summarises his remedies. A new broom approach is always tempting, and getting from where we are to where we would like to be is always expensive, but he may be right that after 70 years of incremental change, mostly for the worse, in the management of this behemoth, a new approach is required.

Certainly, anyone interested in the NHS and its management should read this book. I would be interested to hear what they say about Dr Sarwar's ideas, and hope that the book starts a lively conversation in the corridors of power and in the pubs.

Fantastic book! It is very readable and the author has done a lot of work in collecting the facts and figures to reference his findings. The book provides interesting ideas about the future of our NHS, and insight into where our money is going. It has revealed the hidden privatisation that is occurring, which is in complete contraindication with its creative ethos. Great read for anyone curious as to where our money is going!

A must read. Well, this may change your views. If not it will certainly educate you. It is a great tribute to our Doctors and Nurses but a thought provoking eye opener full of facts and evidence on where our Health Service is going wrong and the people are being misled and let down.

Thank You for writing this helpful book.

I liked the honesty and passion contained in the book, but most of all the bravery and initiative of a qualified Doctor to take that time and trouble to produce this book.

In less than 200 pages Author has explained, the root cause of NHS problems and how to rectify it.
I think it's a must read for all senior members of health care profession

As someone who has experienced the NHS's failings more than most, the system proposed in this book would be a breath of fresh air. It identifies the heart of the issue - an issue I never knew existed - and sets out a way to eradicate it, leaving both the patients and staff the better for it. This book is clearly the result of an enormous amount of research and hard work, and it shows. This is not a clickbait-type exposé, rather it is a well-written, thoroughly researched blueprint of how things must be going forward.

I could not put this book down - a real page turner The author has found out what really happens in the NHS and complements the Staff and sets this in contrast with the real behind the scenes story. Full of interesting facts and figures with a clear way forward to helping the service become the best in the world and the author shows us exactly how this can be achieved. This book contains a successful business model which could be used and worked towards in building a better future.

Printed in Poland
by Amazon Fulfillment
Poland Sp. z o.o., Wrocław